SECOND EDITION

The OTA's Guide to
Writing
SOAP Notes

SECOND EDITION

The OTA's Guide to
Writing
SOAP Notes

Sherry Borcherding, MA, OTR/L
University of Missouri–Columbia
Columbia, MO

Marie J. Morreale, OTR/L, CHT
Rockland Community College
Suffern, NY

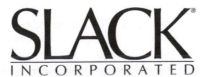
SLACK®
INCORPORATED

Delivering the best in health care information and education worldwide www.slackbooks.com

ISBN-13: 978-1-55642-779-4
ISBN-10: 1-55642-779-4

Published by: SLACK Incorporated
                   6900 Grove Road
                   Thorofare, NJ 08086 USA
                   Telephone: 856-848-1000
                   Fax: 856-853-5991
                   www.slackbooks.com

Contact SLACK Incorporated for more information about other books in this field or about the availability of our books from distributors outside the United States.

Library of Congress Cataloging-in-Publication Data

Borcherding, Sherry.
   The OTA's guide to writing SOAP notes/Sherry Borcherding,
 Marie J. Morreale. -- 2nd ed.
     p. ; cm.
   Includes bibliographical references and index.
   ISBN-13: 978-1-55642-779-4 (alk. paper)
   ISBN-10: 1-55642-779-4 (alk. paper)
   1. Occupational therapy assistants. 2. Medical records.
 3. Medical writing.   I. Morreale, Marie J. II. Title.
   [DNLM: 1. Occupational Therapy--methods. 2. Allied Health
 Personnel. 3. Documentation--methods. 4. Medical Records.
 WB 555 B726o 2007]
 RM735.4.B673 2007
 615.8'515--dc22

                            2006028261

Printed in the United States of America.

Last digit is print number: 10 9   8   7   6   5   4   3   2   1

Dedication

This book is dedicated to all the OT and OTA students we have taught, who have made our work meaningful, and who inspire us with their commitment and caring hearts.

Contents

Acknowledgments

Many people have contributed to this book. First I would like to thank Amy McShane at SLACK Incorporated, who held a vision for this book and its predecessor. Without Amy's vision and persistence, neither of the OTA editions would ever have come into being. I would also like to thank Marie Morreale, who was successful in coauthoring with me from halfway across the country, and Carol Kappel, who was coauthor on the first edition.

I am grateful to Diana Baldwin for teaching me how to teach and for mentoring me in both teaching and writing. Without her loving support I might have taken another path entirely. I am also grateful to Fred Dittrich, to whom I owe my computer skills. Without Fred's intervention, I would still be writing with a pencil. Finally, I would like to thank the occupational therapy students at the University of Missouri who allowed their notes to be used to teach others.

Sherry Borcherding

I would like to thank Ellen Spergel, coordinator of the Occupational Therapy Assistant Program at Rockland Community College, for allowing my life to take a path that I never could have imagined. I appreciate her support of this project and am grateful for her wisdom and guidance regarding OT education. Edward Mechmann and Susan DeMaio also deserve thanks for being so generous with their time at the start of this endeavor. I am truly indebted to Debbie Amini and Kathy Babcock, who are treasured friends and colleagues, for their unending help and support in so many ways throughout this process. Appreciation goes to Mae Eng, Donna Knoebel, Jennifer Krol, Phyllis Mouakad, Michael Nunes, and Lori MacLeod for their expertise regarding different practice areas. My son Michael certainly deserves recognition for helping to resolve my computer issues. Finally, special thanks to my husband Richard. Without his love and support, this book would not have been possible.

Marie J. Morreale

About the Authors

Sherry Borcherding, MA, OTR/L currently serves as a faculty member at University of Missouri–Columbia, a Carnegie Research Extensive University, where she has taught since 1992. She teaches disability awareness, complementary therapy, and a three-semester fieldwork sequence designed to develop critical thinking, clinical reasoning, and documentation skills. She has also taught clinical ethics, frames of reference, psychopathology, loss and disability, long-term care, and wellness. Two of her courses are designated as campus writing courses and one is credentialed for computer and information proficiency. Sherry is frequently invited to present on collaborative learning, peer review, and educational technology.

Sherry graduated with honors from Texas Woman's University with a BS in occupational therapy and went on to complete her master's in special education with special faculty commendation at George Peabody College in Nashville, TN. Following her staff positions in rehabilitation, home health, and pediatrics, she assumed a number of management roles, including Chief Occupational Therapist at East Texas Treatment Center, Director of Occupational Therapy at Mid-Missouri Mental Health Center, and Director of Rehabilitation Services at Transitional Housing Agency. She has also planned, designed, and directed occupational therapy programs at Capital Regional Medical Center in Jefferson City, MO and at Charter Behavioral Health Center in Columbia, MO.

Besides teaching, Sherry consults on quality assurance issues for local behavioral health centers and has a private practice devoted to complementary and alternative therapies. She is certified in CranioSacral Therapy at the techniques level through Upledger Institute and is attuned as a Reiki master. For leisure, Sherry enjoys folk dance, music, and all kinds of three-dimensional art. Her pottery has appeared in several local shows over the past two years.

Marie J. Morreale, OTR/L, CHT has been teaching in the Occupational Therapy Assistant Program at Rockland Community College since 1998. She is part of the adjunct faculty and currently teaches Professional Issues and Documentation, OT Skills, Geriatric Principles, and Advanced OT Skills. Besides making significant contributions to curriculum development, Marie has served as interim program coordinator and has also taught several other courses in the OTA program, including OT Therapeutic Activities and Advanced Therapeutic Activities.

Since graduating Summa Cum Laude from Quinnipiac College (now Quinnipiac University), Marie has worked in a variety of OT practice settings, including inpatient and outpatient rehabilitation, long-term care, adult day care, home health, cognitive rehabilitation, and hand therapy. She also served for several years on a home health Professional Advisory Committee (consulting on quality assurance issues), and has been a Certified Hand Therapist since 1993. In addition, Marie is the author of several online continuing education courses and was selected for *Who's Who Among America's Teachers* in 2003-2004.

When not teaching, Marie is an active member of her church community where she voluntarily chairs various fundraising events and community activities. In addition, Marie is an avid reader and she also enjoys all kinds of domestic and international travel.

Chapter 1

Documenting the Occupational Therapy Process

Introduction

An occupational therapy assistant (OTA) has many roles and responsibilities, including the essential task of writing in the health record. Your professional documentation provides important information and feedback to the occupational therapist and treatment team regarding your clients. Initially, writing in the health record might seem very intimidating to an OTA student or novice practitioner. When you first see an experienced occupational therapist or occupational therapy assistant make an entry in a health record, you might be tempted to think you will never be able to do it. Just the technical language alone can be daunting, and then there is the amazing attention to detail in the client observation, the insightful assessment, and the documentation that just seems to flow from the pen without apparent effort. You may wonder whether you will be able to organize all your client observations, predict what the next steps will be, and record interventions so quickly and professionally. You may also feel apprehensive because the process seems a little foreign to you. Rest assured that the occupational therapy practitioners probably felt the same way as you when they were students.

Professional documentation is a skill, and like any skill, it can be learned. Learning a skill, whether it is downhill skiing, playing the violin, or composing a progress note requires three things of you: 1) instruction, 2) practice, and 3) patience. This manual is designed to get you started with learning and practicing the process. Information is systematically provided on each part of the documentation process, and the worksheets are designed to let you practice each step as you learn it. Use the manual as a workbook. Take time to integrate the information in each section, complete each exercise, and check it against the suggested answers. Reflect and learn from your mistakes, and develop confidence in your documentation abilities.

Overview

Although occupational therapy practitioners write in more than one format, this manual presents a thorough and systematic approach to one form of documentation, the **SOAP** note. SOAP is an acronym for the four parts of an entry into the health record. The letters stand for Subjective, Objective, Assessment, and Plan. You will learn the origins and meanings of these terms in Chapter 2. The format for writing SOAP notes taught in this manual is one that is reimbursable under both managed care and Medicare Part B. While all notes written in occupational therapy practice settings do not have to meet these requirements, the managed care and Medicare Part B standards are the most rigorous. If you learn to meet these strict standards, you are not likely to be denied reimbursement by any third party payer. Current occupational therapy practice is in many ways determined by which services are reimbursable, and documentation of client care is the method by which that service is communicated. This manual will help you to understand the purpose and standards of documentation for various practice settings and different stages of treatment. Many examples of occupational therapy notes are presented. This manual also includes a guide to medical terminology, a brief review of grammar, and a step-by-step guide to the initial evaluation process delineating the roles of the occupational therapist and occupational therapy assistant. Understanding the process will greatly assist you in choosing appropriate client interventions. The Appendix, "Suggestions for Completing the Worksheets," provides "answers" for the worksheets. However, since there are many "right" ways to answer, these must be viewed as suggestions rather than the only correct answers. In actual clinical practice, you will see varied documentation styles among occupational therapy practitioners. Each clinician develops individualized writing skills and a personal repertoire of professional language while still complying with accepted legal and facility standards.

This manual reflects the collaboration of the occupational therapist and occupational therapy assistant and incorporates standards of The American Occupational Therapy Association (AOTA) for education, documentation, and clinical practice. The material presented in this book originally grew out of documentation courses taught to occupational therapy seniors at the University of Missouri–Columbia, a Carnegie Research Intensive University. The material was edited to be more appropriate for clinical practice of OTAs for the first edition of this manual. This second edition combines the original concepts with new material that grew from documentation courses taught to occupational therapy assistant students at Rockland Community College, a unit of the State University of New York. This edition is a collaborative work that reflects the current guidelines for professional documentation and clinical practice. The material has been field tested to be sure it is practical, understandable, and effective in helping you learn both documentation and clinical reasoning skills.

The content of this documentation manual reflects the scope of occupational therapy practice and emphasizes the basis of our services as described in the *Occupational Therapy Practice Framework: Domain and Process* (AOTA, 2002). It also incorporates concepts and guidelines found in

- *Guidelines for Documentation of Occupational Therapy* (AOTA, 2003a)
- *Guidelines for Supervision, Roles, and Responsibilities During the Delivery of Occupational Therapy Services* (AOTA, 2004a)
- *Scope of Practice* (AOTA, 2004b)
- *Occupational Therapy Code of Ethics* (AOTA, 2005b)
- *Standards of Practice for Occupational Therapy* (AOTA, 2005c)

Many occupational therapy assistants were never taught how to write effective notes and had to learn it on the job. They have learned what works in their own situation, but may or may not be prepared to meet the requirements of other practice settings. You will have a head start by using this manual.

Our Professional Language and Focus

Occupational Therapy Practice Framework

The *Occupational Therapy Practice Framework: Domain and Process* (AOTA, 2002), also referred to as the *Framework*, is an important document that embodies the focus and heart of occupational therapy and is a useful resource for documenting professional terminology. The *Framework* describes the domain of occupational therapy as "engagement in occupation to support participation in context or contexts" (AOTA, 2002, p. 610) and holistically delineates best practice for evaluation, intervention, and outcomes. This document presents a client-centered process that centers on enabling individuals to perform desired life activities and meaningful occupations; the *Framework* groups these broad and varied life tasks into **areas of occupation** (AOTA, 2002). The ability to engage in occupation is impacted by many interrelated factors: the client's **performance skills** (in the areas of motor, process, and communication), **performance patterns** (habits, roles, and routines), as well as **activity demands**, internal and external **contexts**, and **client factors** (body structures and body functions) (AOTA, 2002). Your SOAP notes should reflect the professional occupational therapy language and concepts set forth by the *Framework*.

By starting with an **occupational profile**, occupational therapy practitioners are able to determine whether any contextual features, activity demands, or individual client factors need to be addressed, depending on the occupational needs of the client (AOTA, 2002). This allows appropriate goals and interventions to be determined for desired outcomes. The occupational profile is a client-centered approach to gathering information (occupational history, interests, experiences, habits, and patterns of daily living) as well as what the client values, needs, or hopes to gain from the present situation, allowing the client to set priorities for treatment (AOTA, 2002). All this initial data, plus any subsequent changes in the client's status, priorities, interventions, goals, and targeted outcomes, will be recorded in the different types of notes that occupational therapy practitioners write throughout the intervention process.

Influencing Contexts

The *Framework* also describes how clients engage in meaningful occupation in a variety of arenas, or **contexts** (AOTA, 2002). In addition to internal contexts (such as age, culture, values, religion, or developmental stages), a context may be physical (such as home or office), social (such as family or colleague), or virtual (such as the internet) (AOTA, 2002). If your client is being seen in a context such as a hospital or clinic, that is not usual for him, it is important to determine whether or not the skills you are teaching are transferable to his own environment. It is especially important to document how particular contexts relate to the client's condition and may be barriers to occupational performance. For example, a client who has good functional mobility in the hospital may be completely stopped by three steps into a mobile home, a 24-inch door into the bathroom, an old-fashioned bathtub on legs, or lack of an elevator at the job site. A client who lives in a rural area and can no longer drive may not have the option of public transportation for grocery shopping or getting to work. Due to peer pressure, a teenager may refuse to wear leg braces and hand splints or attend counseling. Your documentation should always include relevant contextual issues or problems along with any appropriate intervention or follow-up to address these situations.

Activity demands are interactive. They are most easily thought of in terms of task analysis. The demands of an activity include both what is needed to perform the activity, and how that influences or relates to the client's stated goals.

Underlying Factors

The concepts of **client factors** and **performance skills** are sometimes confused when attempts are made to document a client's abilities and limitations. **Client factors** consist of **body structures** and **body functions,** which refer to the client's anatomy and physiology (AOTA, 2002). For example, an amputation of a limb, a hysterectomy, or a dental extraction would be considered loss of a body structure. An adult with a degenerated joint, scoliosis, or a child born with cleft palate, spina bifida, or club foot all have an impairment in a particular body structure. Body structures provide a physical framework to enable all the body's systems to function, just like a water heater requires a metal container, pipes, nuts, and bolts before it can begin to work.

Some deficits in body structures can be "fixed" permanently or semipermanently (total joint replacement, organ transplant, corrective surgery) or temporarily (dentures, prosthesis, wig). These "corrections" may sometimes necessitate a referral to occupational therapy. For example, intervention may include teaching compensatory dressing techniques following a total hip replacement, improving activity tolerance for a prosthesis, teaching energy conservation following a heart transplant, or improving mood or body image after a mastectomy.

The term *body functions* refers to making the body systems perform their duties, just like the water heater getting turned on and heating the water. The *Framework* groups body functions somewhat similar to the systems of the body, such as neuromusculoskeletal functions, sensory and pain functions, mental functions, etc. (Youngstrom, 2002a). These vital processes include basic life and movement functions such as breathing, righting reactions, reflexes, wound healing, digestion, and immunology. More overt body functions include areas such as strength, pain, the senses, and joint motion. Mental functions encompass cognitive and perceptual skills, and also include affective functions like personality and emotions (AOTA, 2002). If any of these client factors do not limit the client's ability to engage in desired occupational tasks, they do not necessarily need to be assessed or addressed in treatment. However, if a client has issues that do impact function such as poor memory, open wounds, visual neglect, low vision, decreased strength, spasticity, low self-esteem, hallucinations, or anxiety, then these might be relevant client factors to document and target in your interventions.

Performance Skills

Occupational therapy practitioners use professional knowledge to assess the demands or requirements of activities and also to observe and analyze **performance skills**; these are client behaviors and actions grouped into three areas: **motor skills, process skills**, and **communication/interaction skills** (AOTA, 2002). As your client is performing activities, you will examine and document how these skills are performed and consider what factors may impede function. Motor skills consist of actions such as handling objects, mobility, balance, level of energy, and interacting with one's surroundings (AOTA, 2002). For example, you can note your client's ability to carry dishes to the table, reach to get clothes out of the dryer, push a shopping cart, manipulate knitting needles and yarn, bend to pick boxes up from the floor, grip pliers, or stand at the workshop counter for 10 minutes. Process skills consist of focusing and using knowledge and adaptive skills to perform activities, including organizing time and task components (AOTA, 2002). These process skills are evident when you see a child, for example, put away the toys, search for food in the refrigerator, ask for help with homework, choose proper utensils for lunch, attend to the math teacher, or organize a locker.

Communication/interaction skills involve the physical and verbal aspects of communication and relating to others (AOTA, 2002). For example, you can observe the resident request a pain pill, express dissatisfaction about personal life decisions, shake hands or make eye contact with the OTA, speak in a low monotone voice, or share candy with others. You will be recording your professional observations and analysis of client behavior, actions, skills, and underlying client factors in your SOAP notes.

Engaging in Meaningful Occupation

Before we talk about documenting the occupational therapy process, we must differentiate occupational therapy from other healthcare disciplines. Occupational therapists and occupational therapy assistants provide interventions for people who have problems engaging in an **area of occupation**. This is very important to note, because this is what we will document. When documenting occupational therapy services, the focus on ability to engage in occupation is critical for demonstrating the necessity for occupational therapy and for preventing any question of duplication of services (Youngstrom, 2002b). Occupational therapy practitioners in *all* service delivery settings have this common goal of facilitating occupational role performance (Youngstrom, 2002b). It is also important to understand that each third party payer has an interest in different outcomes or areas of occupation, meaning that payers have specific guidelines for what services they allow or consider necessary and will reimburse. This includes the specific type of OT interventions, duration of therapy services, or any special equipment clients may need (i.e., hospital beds, splints, adaptive devices, assistive technology, or customized wheelchairs). Your documentation should reflect those payer interests and requirements as they pertain to the client's condition and needs, living environment/contexts, and realistic expected outcomes. For example, Worker's Compensation will be interested in a client's ability to return to work, Medicare may be concerned about a home care client's ability to safely perform ADL at home, whereas a school district will be concerned about a child's ability to perform educationally related tasks as per the Individualized Education Plan (IEP). The *Framework* describes the following seven areas of occupation (AOTA, 2002):

Activities of Daily Living

Basic or personal activities of daily living (BADL or PADL) are necessary tasks for self-care and personal independence. These are tasks such as bathing, grooming, hygiene, dressing, eating, toileting, sexual activity, sleep, and functional mobility (AOTA, 2002). It is important to consider not just the physical ability to care for self, but also other components, such as cognition or mental health issues that might cause limitations in performance. For example, rather than being unable to perform grooming skills due to a physical factor, a client might fail to notice that his poor hygiene is problematic or he might be depressed and unmotivated to perform self-care. If your services are being reimbursed by Medicare, you will often find yourself writing goals for ADL activities. For children, you will address ADL as developmentally appropriate.

Instrumental Activities of Daily Living

Instrumental activities of daily living (IADL) require more complex problem solving and social skills. IADL include such tasks as money management, cleaning, laundry, child care, driving, shopping, and meal preparation (AOTA, 2002). While these are necessary skills in adulthood, IADL are also important developmental milestones for children and teenagers such as caring for a pet, managing an allowance, babysitting, or using a microwave. Occupational therapy practitioners who work with persons with brain injuries also talk about executive functions that are at issue in frontal lobe damage. Executive functions involve planning, goal setting, and organizational tasks, which impact ability to effectively perform IADL tasks. If your client population has cognitive involvement or mental health problems, you may find that your goals include many IADL activities.

Work

Work includes successfully seeking and carrying out paid employment, as well as participating in volunteer experiences. Work is a primary area of occupation for adults, forms a part of adult identity, and helps to structure one's day. If your services are being reimbursed by Worker's Compensation, you will find that your goals and interventions center around return to work. Other work goals might include injury prevention such as ergonomics, safety education, and the elimination of hazards. If vocational rehabilitation is your payer, you might find instead that your work goals involve helping prepare a client for work that is both meaningful and within the client's capabilities.

Leisure

Leisure activities are those intrinsically rewarding things one does when not obligated to be doing anything else. Leisure is a very important area of occupation, particularly for older people. Leisure and play, especially for adults, are generally considered activities that enhance one's quality of life, and are not usually regarded as being reimbursable goals. However, the performance skills and patterns required to perform leisure activities are transferable to a variety of occupations that are reimbursable. Therefore, leisure is usually approached indirectly in documentation, with a focus on performance skills and patterns. However, in some practice settings such as mental health, it might be appropriate to have leisure-related goals addressing stress management, appropriate use of leisure time, interpersonal, or social components.

Play

In a young child, play can be solitary or social and may consist of organized tasks such as games with rules, or spontaneous activities such as exploratory play. One of the primary occupations for a child is acquiring those skills necessary to progress through age-appropriate developmental milestones, and these skills are acquired through play. When providing occupational therapy to young children, you will often find yourself talking about play in your documentation.

Education

Education is another of the primary occupations of a child. Those activities and skills needed to perform successfully in formal or informal educational settings are unique. Occupational therapy services to children in the educational system are for the purpose of the child performing school-related activities. If you are working in school-based practice, your goals and interventions must relate to behaviors and skills needed in the classroom to be reimbursable. You should also consider the child's ability to engage in extracurricular activities such as music, clubs, and sports. Education for adults encompasses college classes and formal, informal, or personal educational situations such as taking a continuing education seminar for professional needs or personal enrichment (AOTA, 2002).

Social Participation

People, as social beings, need to be able to interact successfully with others and to keep their behavior within the contextual norms of the community, the family, and peer groups. If you are working with clients who have brain injury, developmental disability, or mental health problems, you might find yourself documenting goals and interventions for social participation.

Occupational therapy practitioners are no longer content to see health as the absence of impairment. We now are returning to our roots, and to a view of health that is based on a broader definition—a definition that includes interaction with the environment and satisfaction with overall quality of life.

Skilled Occupational Therapy

Throughout this documentation manual, occupational therapy service is described as **skilled** occupational therapy. This termed originated in Medicare regulations, which define the difference between skilled and nonskilled services. Medicare Part B requirements are being followed in this manual to help insure that your services will not be denied payment. It is important to know that Medicare reimburses those interventions that are identified as skilled and considered reasonable and necessary for the individual's condition. Medicare does not reimburse those services considered nonskilled, not necessary for the client's condition, or if there is no expectation that treatment will be effective (Centers for Medicare and Medicaid Services [CMS], 2005e).

Skilled services have specific criteria. They require professional education, decision making, and highly complex competencies that have a well-defined knowledge base of human functioning and occupational performance. **Nonskilled** services are defined as those that are routine or maintenance types of therapy, both of which could be carried out by nonprofessional personnel or caregivers (CMS, 2005e). This manual emphasizes the necessity of documenting your intervention as **skilled occupational therapy**. This means you must demonstrate the client's potential for functional improvement, or that intervention is necessary for equipment recommendations, establishment of an effective and safe maintenance program, or to address a specific medical need (CMS, 2005e). These criteria justify the services of an OT or OTA. However, Medicare is becoming more stringent in determining where the skill of an occupational therapy practitioner is no longer needed. For example, you may only be reimbursed for one or two occupational therapy sessions for positioning or exercise. In these situations, you are expected to develop the appropriate intervention or prevention program, with follow-up provided by nonskilled personnel or a family member (CMS, 2005e). It is necessary for you to document in a way that differentiates your skill as an occupational therapy practitioner from that of nursing, restorative services, or other rehabilitation disciplines.

Your documentation should demonstrate the level of complexity or sophistication of the services you are providing and reflect treatment appropriate to the individual's condition and rehabilitation potential.

The CMS website (www.cms.hhs.gov) can be a useful resource to review Medicare guidelines and manuals.

Other Reimbursable Services

Safety Concerns

The ability to perform a task must include the ability to do it safely. Intervention strategies targeting safety are usually considered cost-effective services by third party payers because they prevent costly reinjury. Safety concerns include situations such as a high probability of falling; lack of environmental awareness; severe pain; absence of skin sensation; abnormal, aggressive or destructive behaviors; or suicide risk. These all fall within the scope of skilled occupational therapy.

Prevention of Secondary Complications

Preventative interventions are within the scope of skilled occupational therapy if it can be shown that the client has a high risk of developing complications. Secondary complications might include prevention of repetitive strain injuries, progressive joint contractures, fracture nonunion, and skin breakdown or pressure sores. Other prevention programs and strategies might include early intervention programs, drug/alcohol relapse prevention programs, programs for at-risk youth, assessment of ergonomics in the workplace, instruction in joint protection, energy conservation, and provision of wellness programs.

The AOTA website (www.aota.org) contains a section on reimbursement and regulatory policy and is a useful resource to help determine what occupational therapy services are reimbursable.

Roles of the Registered Occupational Therapist and Certified Occupational Therapy Assistant

Occupational therapists (OTs) and occupational therapy assistants (OTAs) have different roles and responsibilities in documenting the occupational therapy intervention process. In AOTA's *Guidelines for Supervision, Roles, and Responsibilities During the Delivery of Occupational Therapy Services* (AOTA, 2004a) and *Standards of Practice for Occupational Therapy* (AOTA, 2005c), the roles and responsibilities of both OTs and OTAs are very specifically delineated regarding documentation and clinical practice. The OTA collaborates with the OT in designing, implementing and assessing occupational therapy services. The OTA may also contribute to documentation at all stages of treatment under the supervision of the OT and concurring with relevant laws and regulations (AOTA, 2004a).

Although these guidelines are considered "best practice," state statutes and licensure laws may differ from the guidelines. The guidelines may also differ from federal laws that delineate mandatory documentation requirements. In addition, reimbursement organizations sometimes specify who would be an approved documenter or service provider for reimbursement purposes. You as an occupational therapy professional are accountable for adhering to the mandatory policies and procedures adopted by state and federal regulatory agencies. However, you will find the standards established by AOTA very useful in interpreting and following regulations.

Types of Notes

Different kinds of notes are written at different stages of the treatment process. Notes also vary according to the type of practice setting. From the first notation in the chart that a referral has been received to the closing lines of the discharge summary, occupational therapy practitioners document the many and varied activities of the intervention process. The specific content of the note, the format and organization of the note, and the time lines required vary according to type of setting, accrediting and regulatory agencies involved, and requirements of third party payers. The contents required for each type of note are described in *Guidelines for Documentation of Occupational Therapy* (AOTA, 2003a). The requirements for the following kinds of notes will be addressed in this manual:

Initial Evaluation Reports

Before beginning treatment, the client is evaluated to determine whether occupational therapy is appropriate for this client, and if so, what kind of therapeutic intervention will be most useful. The occupational therapist directs the initial evaluation process, documents the results, and establishes the intervention plan, although the occupational therapy assistant can contribute to this process (AOTA, 2005c). Each practice setting or facility has its own way of evaluating a client. A mental health center, for example, may not do the same kind of an initial evaluation as a public school or a skilled nursing facility. Initial evaluations are usually documented on specific forms provided by the setting, but may also be done in a SOAP format.

Contact Notes

Each time an intervention is provided by the occupational therapy practitioner, notation is made of what occurred. Contacts may also include pertinent telephone conversations and meetings with the client, family/caregiver, other professionals, or service providers. In some settings, each treatment session is documented in the health record using a contact note. In other settings, the occupational therapy practitioner keeps a log or makes notes to himself for use later in writing progress notes, but no formalized contact note is required. Contact notes can be written in many different formats, but in this manual the SOAP format will be taught.

Progress Notes

At the end of a specified period of time, a progress note is written. The occupational therapy practitioner records the client's progress toward goals and details any changes made in the intervention plan. Different practice settings vary regarding time periods for reporting, but progress notes are usually written weekly or monthly. Progress notes may also be written in different formats, but will be taught in a SOAP format in this manual.

Reevaluation Notes

The OT directs and documents the reevaluation that is part of the occupational therapy intervention process and modifies the intervention plan according to the client's needs. The OTA may contribute to this reevaluation process (AOTA, 2005c). Some settings require a formal reevaluation report. For example, in a practice setting where managed care is involved, a client may need to be reevaluated in order to be recertified for treatment after the number of initially allocated visits are completed.

Transition Notes

Transition notes are written when a client is transferring from one service setting to another, such as from acute care to rehabilitation or from rehabilitation to skilled nursing, within the same service delivery system (AOTA, 2003a). Transition notes insure that the client's intervention plan remains intact through the move, and that services that have already been provided are not duplicated. The transition plan is the responsibility of the OT, but the OTA can contribute to this process (AOTA, 2005c).

Discharge or Discontinuation Notes

At the end of treatment, a discharge or discontinuation note is written to describe changes in the client's ability to engage in meaningful occupation as a result of occupational therapy intervention. The discontinuation plan is directed and documented by the OT, but the OTA may contribute to this process (AOTA, 2005c). Discharge notes summarize the course of treatment, progress toward goals, status at the time of discharge, any adaptive equipment or splints provided, any home program that may have been recommended, and any other recommendations, referrals, or follow-up required. Some settings will provide a specific form for the discharge note and other facilities may use the same form that was used for the evaluation. For purposes of this manual, we will use a SOAP format.

Names and other details have been fabricated in this manual to protect the confidentiality of those people who receive our services. In a note that says "Mr. D. was seen in his home..." please understand that he is being called "Mr. D." for purposes of confidentiality. If you were writing a note in his health record, you would use his whole name and any other required identifying information. Also, realize that each client has unique circumstances and needs. Although this manual provides sound guidelines for documenting occupational therapy practice, you must always use your clinical judgment when treating clients and documenting in the medical record.

New in This Edition

The second edition of *The OTA's Guide to Writing SOAP Notes* is based on the *Occupational Therapy Practice Framework: Domain and Process* (AOTA, 2002) and AOTA's more recent documents: the *Guidelines for Documentation of Occupational Therapy* (AOTA, 2003a), *Guidelines for Supervision, Roles, and Responsibilities During the Delivery of Occupational Therapy Services* (AOTA, 2004a), *Scope of Practice* (AOTA, 2004b), *Occupational Therapy Code of Ethics* (AOTA, 2005b), and *Standards of Practice for Occupational Therapy* (AOTA, 2005c). The second edition includes a brief discussion of health record management, billing codes, and HIPAA. More information on the mechanics of documentation, medical terminology, and the roles of the OT and OTA during the initial evaluation, intervention, and outcome process has also been included. In addition, the examples used in the text and the worksheets are more diverse, with increased examples from mental health, hand therapy, and pediatric practice settings. Some chapters have been reorganized to make the material easier to understand. Other chapters have been added or expanded to address spelling and grammar, special situations, improving observation skills, understanding the initial evaluation process, and selecting appropriate interventions. Worksheets have also been added and revised for optimal learning and practice.

Conclusion

The following two worksheets will help you practice using the *Framework* terminology to record your observations. Then, in the following chapters, you will be introduced to the health record and to the specifics of your documentation in the record. Professional documentation pulls together all your observation skills, clinical reasoning, and knowledge of occupational therapy. There will be ample explanation and opportunity for practice so that you will systematically acquire the appropriate documentation skills. Eventually, *you* will be the occupational therapy assistant we talked about in the beginning paragraph whose documentation was so amazing to the beginning student.

Worksheet 1-1
Using the *Occupational Therapy Practice Framework*

Observe someone making an object out of clay or another craft project. Use terminology from the *Occupational Therapy Practice Framework* and list 10 specific performance skills or client factors that you observe or assess during this activity. Try to describe, qualify, or quantify levels of performance.

Activity Observed: _____

Example:

Process Skill: Attends well to task

Client factor: Has good range of motion in both hands

1.

2.

3.

4.

5.

6.

7.

8.

9.

10.

Worksheet 1-2
Occupational Therapy Practice Framework—More Practice

Observe someone performing a cooking task such as making tea, a sandwich, or can of soup. Use terminology from the *Occupational Therapy Practice Framework* and list 10 specific performance skills or client factors that you observe or assess during this activity. Try to describe, qualify, or quantify levels of performance.

Activity Observed: _____

Example:

    Motor skill: Coordinates use of both hands well when using can opener

    Client factor: Able to hear whistling tea kettle

1.

2.

3.

4.

5.

6.

7.

8.

9.

10.

Chapter 2

The Health Record

Definition and Purpose

The medical record is a compilation of unique personal and medical information relating to a client (Fremgen, 2006). It is also sometimes called the health record as healthcare shifts to programs or models oriented toward wellness and prevention. You will see both terms used throughout this book. The medical (or health) record is a **legal document** that includes the client's past and present health information, current diagnosis, course of treatment, and related correspondence (Fremgen, 2006). The primary purpose of the record is the exchange of information among a client's healthcare providers in order to determine problems, concerns, and strengths, plan and record treatment, substantiate care, and fulfill legal documentation requirements (Iyer, 2002). You, as an OTA, will use the record frequently to obtain and record essential client information.

Although the health record is the physical property of the healthcare facility that furnishes the client's care, the client owns the recorded information (Iyer, 2002). Therefore, you should realize that individuals do have a right to review and obtain a copy of their records (including what you have written in OT). However, there are some exceptions or circumstances that may limit access. For example, a physician may use professional discretion to determine if a client with mental health issues would be harmed by reviewing his or her own health record (Fremgen, 2006). In order to obtain their records, patients usually have to write a formal request and may also be charged for the copying costs. Your facility will have policies regarding this process.

Third party payers may require health record documentation to substantiate claims for reimbursement. In those cases, generally the original paperwork stays in the chart and copies are sent or faxed. Each facility establishes policies to delineate which departments or personnel are responsible for sending out records to clients, physicians, other professionals, or third party payers. All staff must be very careful when using fax machines, copiers, and e-mail to avoid breaches of confidentiality to unintended recipients. In limited instances, original paperwork such as evaluations or progress reports might need to be sent to the physician for his/her signature and then the signed original gets sent back to the facility. This may be necessary in outpatient settings to follow through on verbal orders or to certify for Medicare that the patient requires skilled services and the physician approves the plan of care. For these situations, facility policies must be strictly adhered to and a copy must also remain in the chart. Privacy laws regulate the disclosure of medical information. **Never give out or send any health records or client information without knowing the exact policies and procedures in your facility**.

Like so many other aspects of healthcare, the health record is rapidly undergoing vast changes as we move further into the information age. As medicine advanced, so did the complexity and detail of the record. A profession, now called Health Information Management, was created to oversee the record.

Storing and Retaining Health Records

There are specific legal guidelines for storing, managing, and retaining health records. Each facility establishes its own policies and procedures to comply with this process and the OTA must follow these protocols. Active health records may be held in a school or agency's administrative office, or at a facility's central location (i.e., nurse's station), or stay within each discipline's department, such as within outpatient occupational or physical therapy departments (Sames, 2005). In hospitals, where records are normally held at the nurse's station, records may proceed with the client to other areas of the facility, such as the radiology department or OT clinic (Sames, 2005).

Normally records must remain and be completed on-site and not be taken home to review or complete documentation. However, an occupational therapy practitioner working in home care or traveling within a school district might be allowed to keep a partial or temporary working copy of records while the original stays within the agency. It is essential to always follow HIPAA guidelines and know your facility's policies.

To ensure privacy of active or inactive health information, keep records in a secure location such as a locked file cabinet, drawer, storage unit, or office rather than leaving them open on your desk, treatment table, or mat, or visible on a computer screen where they might inadvertently be seen by others (Sames, 2005). Volunteers, visitors, or other employees such as housekeeping, maintenance, secretarial staff, or other disciplines may have valid reasons to enter your office or treatment area so you should manage records properly at all times to protect confidentiality. In addition, be especially careful when you are writing things down during a treatment session or conversing about clients in public areas. You must ensure that other people cannot inappropriately see or hear the confidential information.

Individual states mandate the specific minimum time periods for retaining medical records for minors and adults, including OT documentation (Fremgen, 2006). As patients are discontinued or charts become old, records may eventually be moved to another storage area, placed on microfilm, or after the state time requirements are met, might even be destroyed due to storage space limitations (Fremgen, 2006). In this case, it is essential that all records be destroyed properly (meaning incineration or shredding), so that no one else can ever read the confidential health information (Sames, 2005). Realize that any other paperwork containing confidential client information not normally kept in the chart (such as any personal notations, drafts, or working copies used for day to day OT treatment), must also be properly destroyed rather than just discarded in a garbage pail (Sames, 2005). Most departments have shredders or designated locked bins readily available for this purpose.

Advances in technology have created widespread use of computerized healthcare information systems. Information can now be entered and obtained from different locations and means such as wireless devices, the telephone, and internet. Electronic documentation also allows people in different departments to review client data at the same time, such as medical orders or lab results. However, although the electronic health record makes records easily accessible, organized, and legible, it also creates problems such as security and privacy issues, computer downtime, inaccurate entry, or accidental destruction of information (Iyer, 2002).

HIPAA

In 1996, Congress passed the Health Insurance Portability and Accountancy Act (HIPAA), which established national standards to manage and protect the privacy and security of an individual's health information. HIPAA also defined standards for clients' right to understand and control the use of their own health information (United States Department of Health and Human Services [USDHHS], 2003).

The Privacy Rule required compliance by April 14, 2003 (with a 1-year extension for small health plans) and defined regulations for the use and disclosure of **protected health information** (PHI), which is defined as "individually identifiable health information" (USDHHS, 2003, p.3). A major part of the Privacy Rule is the "minimum necessary" standard (USDHHS, 2003, p.10), which states that only the minimum amount of protected health information must be requested or disclosed to accomplish the intended purpose. Facilities and individuals providing health and medical services and who transmit health information electronically (i.e., claims, referral authorization requests, payment), are considered a covered entity under this law (USDHHS, 2003). Occupational therapy practitioners come under this category and must adhere to the HIPAA regulations.

The Problem Oriented Medical Record

The problem oriented medical record (POMR) was introduced in the 1960s by Lawrence Weed, a physician who wanted to provide a more client-centered approach to the structure of the medical record (Kiger, 2003). Weed regarded the record as being arranged for the convenience of staff, rather than ordered for the highest good of the client. He suggested that the record be organized into four distinct sections:

1. A database containing the patient's history and physical evaluations by all disciplines, lab results, etc.

2. A list of the client's problems.

3. An interdisciplinary treatment plan, developed by all the clinicians involved with the client.

4. Progress notes written in chronological order, regardless of discipline.

This format avoids the fragmentation of the source oriented record because it focuses holistically on the client's problems and demonstrates the progress toward solving those problems (Kiger, 2003). It eliminates the need to search the chart to see what each discipline has to say about a particular area of concern. The progress notes are integrated, instead of organized by discipline, so that all the information regarding what has happened for/to the client on a particular day is in one place. Therefore, it is easy for any member of the healthcare team to read progress notes for the last 24 hours and know all the current information without having to search several sections of the chart for the necessary information.

As a part of the more client-centered approach to documentation, Weed recommended that the progress note include the client's own perception of the situation (which had heretofore been considered irrelevant) and be organized into four sections. These four sections included:

S (Subjective): the client's perception of the treatment being received, the progress, limitations, needs and problems. Normally the subjective section of the note is brief. However, in an occupational therapy initial evaluation note, the "S" might be longer because it contains the information obtained by occupational therapy practitioners in the initial interview.

O (Objective): the health professional's observations of the treatment being provided. In an occupational therapy initial evaluation note, this section also contains of all the measurable, quantifiable, and observable data that the OT determines should be collected. In an evaluation, the first two sections form the database from which the OT, with contributions from the OTA, develops a problem list and treatment plan. Some facilities have combined the first two sections into a composite category called **data**, and have adapted Weed's *SOAP* notes into *DAP* notes (Data, Assessment, Plan). For the purposes of this manual, the two discrete sections will continue to be used.

A (Assessment): the health professional's interpretation of the meaning of the events reported in the objective section. This section includes the client's functional limitations, along with expectations of the client's ability to benefit from therapy (sometimes called *rehabilitation potential*). In an initial evaluation, the OT, with feedback from the OTA, will determine and include the problem list, which is one of the key elements of the POMR method of charting. In a progress note, the assessment component explicitly states progress or the lack of progress. In a POMR, each progress note is linked to a problem from the client's problem list. That problem is stated at the beginning of the note.

P (Plan): what the health professional plans to do next to continue with the goals and objectives in the intervention plan. In an occupational therapy initial evaluation, this section contains the OT's intervention plan, including the anticipated frequency and duration of treatment.

For nearly 30 years, Weed's system was popular in hospitals and rehabilitation centers. Gradually, however, many facilities have returned to a more source oriented medical record, divided into sections for each discipline. The discipline's information is in chronological order within each section, making it easy for someone to locate information for a select discipline. However, it is more difficult to find integrated information for specific items or problems due to the size of the chart and lack of an index (Kiger, 2003). Even so, the SOAP format of progress notes has remained popular in facilities that use source oriented or integrated formats rather than the POMR.

Remember that SOAP is simply a format—an outline for organizing information. Any note can be written in this format, although some notes lend themselves to it better than others. For example, the OT, with contributions from the OTA, could write an initial assessment in a SOAP format, or a reassessment, progress note, or a discharge summary. An initial assessment written in this format can be quite lengthy, as it will contain an occupational profile, a summary of functional problems, long- and short-term goals, prior level of functioning, and the beginning intervention plan. OTs and OTAs often use the SOAP format to record client interventions for contact or treatment notes. Remember that all medical record documentation must be in accordance with facility and legal standards. The SOAP format is an alternative to narrative notes, which tend to be disorganized and subjective. It forces the writer to look at all four aspects of the intervention session, and to present the information contained in the note in an organized way. A more detailed discussion of each section of the note will follow in Chapters 5 through 9.

Users and Uses of the Health Record

The health record is a communication tool, and thus has many different uses and users. As an OTA, it is important to consider all your different audiences when you make an entry in the client's record.

Client Care Management

The record is one method the treatment team uses to communicate with each other about the day-to-day aspects of a client's care. Other occupational therapy practitioners in your department or other members of the treatment team will read your notes in order to coordinate care. The OT, with contributions from the OTA, will document the results of the OT evaluation in the health record and establish the intervention plan. The OT and OTA will then collaborate to implement treatment, record the client's progress toward established goals, and advise other team members of the occupational therapy plan for continuing care. This communication is extremely important to the treatment team. In a situation where occupational therapy is provided 7 days per week, one occupational therapy practitioner may not be providing all of the client's care and may depend upon the treatment notes to find out what treatment was provided in his or her absence.

Reimbursement

The health record is the source document for what services were provided, and thus, for what OT services may be billed. It is used in billing to substantiate reimbursement claims. For example, if a question arises about the duration and frequency of interventions provided, the record would be the source document used to answer that question. Often, in managed care, the initial evaluation and periodic progress reports must be submitted in order to obtain preauthorization for subsequent therapy sessions.

The Legal System

The health record is a legal document that substantiates what occurred during a client's illness and course of treatment. If you as an OTA have to appear in court to testify, you will be very glad that your documentation is clear and thorough. Sometimes court cases will occur years after the event or intervention that is being contested and you may not even remember the client or the event. What you have written in the health record should provide you with the information you need to testify. Therapy records may be subpoenaed for many reasons, including cases involving Worker's Compensation, malpractice, personal injury lawsuits, or child, spousal, or elder abuse.

Quality Improvement (QI)

Most facilities have a Quality Improvement (QI) Committee whose duty it is to oversee the appropriateness and adequacy of the care that is being provided. This committee is in charge of finding and solving problems in client care. The health record is one of the primary sources of information used in the QI process.

Research and Evidence Based Practice

The record is also used to provide data for medical research and evidence based practice. Researchers might use individual data specific to that client or aggregate data where no client name is attached to the data. In either case, the source document is often the health record, under the security regulations of HIPAA.

Accreditation

Accrediting agencies such as the Commission on Accreditation of Rehabilitation Facilities (CARF) and the Centers for Medicare and Medicaid Services (CMS) review your notes to ascertain whether the extent and quality of services provided by your facility and/or your department meet the standards of care set by the accrediting agency. If your facility is found not in compliance, accreditation may be withdrawn. For example, CMS accredits facilities that bill Medicare for services provided. If the facility does not meet CMS standards, all claims made by that facility for Medicare services (including occupational therapy) will be denied. The health record is one of the primary sources used during an accreditation visit.

Education

The record may be used as a teaching tool. A student uses the health record to gain information about clients and learn about quality and appropriate occupational therapy intervention, in accord with the security regulations of HIPAA.

Public Health

The record is used to identify and to document the incidence of certain diseases, such as tuberculosis or HIV and outbreaks of contagious illness within a facility. In addition, the record is used to report vital statistics (births, deaths), substantiate and report child, spousal, or elder abuse, and provide statistics for epidemiology (Fremgen, 2006).

Utilization Management

In a hospital setting, the Utilization Review Committee is responsible for determining how services in the facility are being utilized; i.e., what kinds of clients are being seen and what kind of care is being provided, and whether these are appropriate to the mission of the facility.

Business Development

Management teams use the information contained in the record to review, plan, and market the services provided by the facility. For example, are enough cases of eating disorders being admitted to open a special eating disorders unit?

The Client

Another significant user is the client himself. When you are writing in the record, always remember that the client owns the information in his own health record and may choose to exercise his right to read what you have written.

Billing Codes

Diagnosis and billing codes are used by physicians and other healthcare providers when submitting claims for reimbursement. You, as an OTA, will need to align the appropriate codes to your client's condition and interventions. Facilities establish specific procedures for the billing process and will provide you with the necessary resources.

CPT Codes

The mandatory Healthcare Common Procedure Coding System (HCPCS) enables physicians and other healthcare providers to use common language and standardized codes. These codes allow data collection and identification of products and services (CMS, 2005f). The system consists of two parts: Level I and Level II. Level I consists of five-digit codes called Current Procedural Terminology (CPT) codes, which are maintained by the American Medical Association (AMA) and are updated annually (CMS, 2005f). Some codes are based on time (broken into 15-minute time periods) and others are "procedures," which are billed at the same amount regardless of how much time is used. Some codes are mutually exclusive and cannot be billed together (CMS, 2005a). For example, an OT evaluation (an untimed procedure) may not be billed along with a manual muscle test, since the manual muscle test is considered a part of the evaluation (Gennerman, 2005). Also, there are clear billing rules regarding treating more than one client at a time or two disciplines performing a joint treatment to one client (CMS, 2005a).

The Level II codes are maintained by CMS and are alphanumeric, consisting of one letter and four digits (CMS, 2005f). These reflect codes for products and services provided outside of a physician's office such as supplies, durable medical equipment, prosthetics, and orthotics. No trade names are specified within these codes (CMS, 2005b).

Many of these codes are applicable to occupational therapy, reflecting the different types of interventions we provide. However, rather than fully utilizing all the options available, Gennerman (2005) suggests that occupational therapy practitioners often tend to use only a limited variety of intervention codes (such as those for therapeutic exercise, therapeutic activities, training in self-care, home management, or safety), in part because agencies might only provide a predetermined code list. Code books may be purchased from various sources, and codes are also published on the CMS website.

International Classification of Diseases Codes

The International Classification of Diseases (ICD) was developed by the World Health Organization (WHO). ICD-9-CM refers to the 9th version of the ICD codes, which are currently in use in the United States for reporting diseases (morbidity) (WHO, 2006). The WHO has also established ICD-10, which the United States has been using since 1999 to report mortality (WHO, 2006). The ICD-9-CM codes are three-, four-, or five-digit codes that classify diagnoses, symptoms, or complaints. These codes are used for healthcare statistics and billing and are very specific in classification. For example, a fracture is coded by the particular bone, part of bone, and whether it is a closed or open fracture. Code books may be purchased from various sources, including the US Government Printing Office. Also, free training in basic ICD-9 coding is available from the CMS learning website at http://www.cms.hhs.gov/medlearn/therapy.

Writing in the Record

Since the health record is not only a communication tool during the client's hospital stay, but is also the source document for financial, legal, and clinical accountability, the record should indicate the following:
- What services were provided, where, and when.
- What happened and what was said.
- How the client responded to the service provided.
- Why skilled occupational therapy services were needed rather than the services of an aide or family member.

Before you write anything in the record, make these assumptions:
- Someone else will have to read and understand what I write because I may be sick or out of town the next time this client needs to be treated.
- This entry I am about to make will be the one scrutinized by a CMS review team or managed care representative. If I were a funding source, would I want to pay for the OT services I am about to record?
- This entry I am about to make will be subpoenaed and scrutinized by attorneys. If I were called upon to testify, will I be able to recall pertinent client information based on this record?
- My client will exercise his right to read this record.

As mentioned in Chapter 1, it is important that your documentation reflects the different requirements, time frames, and outcomes that third party payers insist on. With a Medicare client, you will normally discuss activities of daily living (ADL) and write goals for self-care activities as Medicare looks for **functional** improvement. It is not enough to simply indicate that the client is working towards a goal of increasing shoulder range of motion. You must indicate what this increased motion will enable the client to do, such as get food out of the refrigerator or put on a shirt. With a Workers' Compensation case, your documentation will be oriented toward the client's return to work or prevention of a costly injury. For example, a computer programmer who has carpal tunnel syndrome may benefit from ergonomic education, adaptive equipment, and a splint in order to alleviate symptoms for work tasks and prevent surgery. With home care, your documentation may focus on your elderly client being unable to leave home to receive services or that you provided education to the caregiver regarding safety issues. If your documentation states that your client is shopping at the mall or driving to the grocery store, then payment will likely be denied as this indicates the client is not really homebound. With a child, you will need to write about developmental needs or educationally related services identified in the Individualized Education Program (IEP). Thus, your notes must indicate how your intervention facilitates the child's performance in school.

Also remember these facts when planning to write in the health record:

- Accuracy is your best protection against problems. You cannot be accurate if you wait too long to record what happened.
- A note in the health record will be a reflection of your professional identity and abilities as well as a reflection of your department and occupational therapy as a profession.
- No activity or contact is ever considered a service that has been provided until a clinical entry is in the record. In terms of legal and fiscal accountability, "If it isn't written, it didn't happen."

Here are some helpful hints on writing notes:

- Avoid generalities.
- Be as concise as possible without leaving out pertinent data.
- Report behavior objectively and avoid judgments except in assessing your data.
- Be sparse with technical jargon that may be unfamiliar to the reader.
- Be careful when copying or writing down information to avoid errors.

The Mechanics of Documentation

There are a few "rules" that must be followed when writing in the health record:

1. **Always use waterproof black ink**. After a certain period of time, health records are microfilmed, and black ink is the only color that microfilms adequately.

2. **Never use correction fluid or correction tape**. Using correction fluid or correction tape in a health record is considered illegally altering the record. The health record is a legal document that must always stand as originally written.

3. **Correct errors**. If you make an error in the health record, draw one line through it, then above the mistake date and sign your initials (Kettenbach, 2004). Do not attempt to change a word or phrase by writing over it or squeezing in additional words.

mm 8/10/06

Pt. able to dress lower body with ~~verbal cues~~ min Ⓐ using a reacher.

In a POMR, if you inadvertently write your note in the wrong client's chart, draw a single line through the entire entry and write "wrong chart" beside it with your signature.

If you need to add something after you have written and signed your note, write an addendum with the current date and time.

4. **Do not erase**. This is also considered illegally altering the record and is another reason that waterproof ink should be used.

5. **Do not leave blank spaces or lines**. Draw a horizontal line through the center of blank spaces. This prevents the record from being altered at a later date.

6. **Be sure all required data is present**. The *Guidelines for Documentation of Occupational Therapy* (AOTA, 2003a) specify the contents for each type of OT note such as an evaluation report, contact note, or discharge report. This information will be addressed in other chapters of this manual. Make certain that your documentation contains all the required basic information such as the facility name, department name, and type of note (AOTA, 2003a). For source oriented medical records, this is usually included as a heading at the top of each page. The information might already be preprinted on your facility's forms, perhaps with a different form for each type of note. Here is an example:

XYZ Home Health Care Agency
Occupational Therapy Department
Progress Note

In addition, you must always write your client's first and last name on each piece of documentation along with any applicable health record number or identification number. In some settings, this information is stamped using an addressograph card. This identifying information will ensure that documentation is placed in the correct chart if papers accidentally get mixed up or if loose papers fall out of charts. Always check with your facility, but generally, the client's name is written as last name, comma, then first name (Doe, Jane). Be especially careful to avoid clerical errors with record numbers, different spellings of similar sounding names (Jean, Gene, Jeanne), or with unfamiliar or complex ethnic names (Coffman-Kadish, 2003).

7. **Sign and date every note**. Remember, it is absolutely critical that you date and sign every note. The notes written by an OTA and students may also need to be cosigned by a supervising OT when the agency or state regulations require this (AOTA, 2003a). The standard of signature is first name, middle initial if available, last name, and credentials. Some settings require a printed name and credentials beneath the signature (Olson, 2004). In addition, some facilities require that you document the time of day that occupational therapy services were provided or phone calls were made.

8. **Be concise**. In today's healthcare system, busy professionals are often pressed for time. They will appreciate being able to read what you have written in the shortest time possible, and your own time for documentation will also be limited under today's productivity standards.

9. **Use appropriate terminology for the recipients of services**. When referring to the persons who use occupational therapy services, the terms client, patient, consumer, resident, veteran, participant, individual, student, teacher, child, caregiver, employer, or family may be used. Please use the term that is considered most respectful and appropriate for your practice setting.

10. **Be prudent in using abbreviations**. Use only the abbreviations that are approved by your facility and do not make up abbreviations. This will be further addressed in Chapter 3.

11. **Refer to yourself, the clinician, in the third person** (Kettenbach, 2004). Avoid referring to yourself with the words "I" or "me." For example, instead of recording, *"Child attempted to bite me,"* write, *"Child attempted to bite clinician."* As another example, instead of writing, *"I instructed the client in dressing skills,"* write, *"COTA instructed the client in dressing skills."* It is even better to focus on the client, rather than the clinician in your note (Kettenbach, 2004), such as *"Client was instructed in dressing skills."*

12. **Use proper spelling and grammar**. Facilities have different styles of organizing and writing information. Some facilities will allow you to use sentence fragments or incomplete sentences and you will notice this in some of the examples in this book. Other facilities may have a more formal style and may insist on complete sentences. Follow the style used in your particular facility and always use proper spelling and grammar. This will be addressed further in Chapter 4.

13. **Notes continued**. If your note for a particular entry does not fit on one page, at the end write: (cont.). Then, on the next page that you resume writing the same note, write the date and: (OT note cont.).

14. **Always adhere to ethical and legal guidelines**. Keep abreast of laws, regulatory guidelines, facility policies, and AOTA's documents concerning both the delivery of occupational therapy services and documentation. This includes antidiscrimination and privacy laws, issues regarding reimbursement, fraud and abuse, certification, continuing competency, supervision, scope of practice, and other pertinent issues.

15. **Always be truthful and objective**. The information you record should never be misleading, fabricated, or falsified (AOTA, 2005b). Don't guess at or embellish information, be careful to avoid personal complaints, and do not judge, criticize, or blame other employees in your note (Kettenbach, 2004).

16. **Write legibly**. Remember that other professionals or insurance companies will be reading and reviewing your notes. Pharmacists, therapists, and other healthcare workers often complain that they are unable to decipher prescriptions and medical documentation because the doctor's (or other health professional's) handwriting is so bad. This can possibly lead to serious errors. It is essential that your notes be understandable in order to communicate effectively and avoid mistakes.

As you now realize by completing this chapter, your occupational therapy documentation serves many purposes. When writing in the health record, all occupational therapy practitioners and students are obliged to adhere to specific professional, legal, and ethical standards (AOTA, 2005a). Follow the guidelines listed in this chapter for the basic rules of documentation. The subsequent chapters and worksheets will then help you to develop effective communication skills and improve clinical reasoning for documentation. Remain patient, keep practicing, and remember that someday soon your SOAP notes will be an important component of your client's health record.

Chapter 3

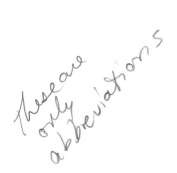

Using Medical Terminology

Healthcare professionals are often pressed for time but are still obligated to complete documentation within established time frames. The use of symbols and abbreviations can certainly help to save time, but the OTA must use them very carefully and judiciously. Remember that your notes may be read by someone who knows little about occupational therapy and who will determine whether or not to pay for your services. In addition, other disciplines such as teachers, aides, or quality improvement personnel may not be familiar with certain medical jargon and may have difficulty interpreting the information. It is prudent to be sure that the person reading your notes is able to understand what you have written. Your facility will be able to furnish a list of the abbreviations it allows so that the abbreviations and symbols that you use will be validated if there is a question. **Do not** make up your own abbreviations, and do not use any abbreviation that is not on your facility's approved list. Remember, it is **permitted** to use abbreviations, but it is not necessary. You are permitted to write out any word instead of shortening it. In this manual, you will find that some practice settings use more abbreviations and symbols than others.

The Joint Commission on the Accreditation of Healthcare Organizations (JCAHO), which accredits hospitals and other healthcare facilities, does not maintain a list of acceptable abbreviations and symbols for use in documentation, although it does maintain a list of those that are prohibited (JCAHO, 2005). **JCAHO encourages clinicians to write out words rather than relying on abbreviations and symbols**. When in doubt, refer to the JCAHO website at www.jcaho.org. A nonprofit organization called The Institute for Safe Medication Practices (ISMP) has also compiled a list of abbreviations and symbols that are prone to error and miscommunication (ISMP, 2005). This list, which includes more than the required JCAHO standards, can be found on the ISMP website (www.ismp.org).

In order to maintain uniformity and maintain clarity in the health record, each healthcare facility establishes a list of approved abbreviations and symbols that clinicians may use in documentation. For purposes of using this manual, the list of abbreviations in Table 3-1 will be permitted. Realize that this list is not all-inclusive and that there are entire books devoted to medical abbreviations. As an OTA, you will certainly encounter other commonly used and acceptable anatomical abbreviations that are not specifically delineated in this manual, such as those for specific nerves, spinal segments, ligaments, and muscles, e.g., flexor carpi ulnaris (FCU). Also, this manual cannot possibly include all the specialized medical or rehabilitation tests and terms that might be specific to your particular practice area. As healthcare evolves, medical terms and abbreviations can become obsolete and be replaced by new terminology. Keep current by joining professional associations and reading professional books and journals. Again, always check with your facility regarding acceptable abbreviations appropriate for your work setting.

Table-3-1

Abbreviations and Symbols

Ⓐ	assistance	CAD	coronary artery disease	DIP	distal interphalangeal joint
ā	before	CAT	computerized axial tomography	DJD	degenerative joint disease
AA	Alcoholics Anonymous				
AAROM	active assisted range of motion	CBC	complete blood count	DM	diabetes mellitus
abd	abduction	CCU	coronary (cardiac) care unit	DME	durable medical equipment
add	adduction	CGA	contact guard assist	DNR	do not resuscitate
ADD	attention deficit disorder	CHF	congestive heart failure	D.O.	doctor of osteopathic medicine
ADHD	attention deficit hyperactivity disorder	CHI	closed head injury	DOA	date of admission; dead on arrival
ADL	activity of daily living	CHT	Certified Hand Therapist	DOB	date of birth
ad lib.	as desired			DOE	dyspnea on exertion
AE	above elbow	cm	centimeter	DPT	doctor of physical therapy
AFO	ankle-foot orthosis	CMC	carpometacarpal		
AIDS	acquired immunodeficiency syndrome	CNS	central nervous system	Dr.	doctor
		CO_2	carbon dioxide	DRG	diagnostic related group
AK	above knee	C/O	complains of		
AKA	above knee amputation	cont.	continued; continue	DRUJ	distal radioulnar joint
		COPD	chronic obstructive pulmonary disease	DTR	deep tendon reflex
ALS	amyotrophic lateral sclerosis			DVT	deep vein thrombosis
		COPM	Canadian Occupational Performance Measure	Dx	diagnosis
a.m., AM	morning			ECG	electrocardiogram
AMA	against medical advice, American Medical Association	COTA	certified occupational therapy assistant	ECHO	echocardiogram
				ECT	electroconvulsive therapy
AMB	ambulation	CP	cerebral palsy		
amt.	amount	CPM	continuous passive motion	EEG	electroencephalogram
ant	anterior			EKG	electrocardiogram
AP	anterior-posterior	CPR	cardiopulmonary resuscitation	EMG	electromyogram
appt.	appointment			ENT	ear, nose, throat
AROM	active range of motion	CRPS	complex regional pain syndrome	EOB	edge of bed
ASAP	as soon as possible			ER	external rotation; emergency room
ASHD	arteriosclerotic heart disease	CSF	cerebrospinal fluid		
		CST	craniosacral therapist	e-stim	electrical stimulation
Ⓑ	bilateral	CT	computed tomography	etc.	etcetera
BADL	basic activity of daily living	CTD	cumulative trauma disorder	ETOH	ethyl alcohol
				eval.	evaluation
BE	below elbow	CTR	carpal tunnel release	exam	examination
BK	below knee	CTRS	certified therapeutic recreation specialist	ext.	extension
BKA	below knee amputation			F	Fahrenheit; Fair (muscle strength grade of 3)
		CTS	carpal tunnel syndrome		
BM	bowel movement				
BP	blood pressure	CVA	cerebrovascular accident	f	female
BRP	bathroom privileges			F.A.C.P.	fellow of the American College of Physicians
c̄	with	CXR	chest x-ray		
C	Celsius; centigrade	d	day	F.A.C.S.	fellow of the American College of Surgeons
C&S	culture and sensitivity	Ⓓ	dependent		
CA	carcinoma; cancer	D&C	dilation and curettage	FBS	fasting blood sugar
CABG	coronary artery bypass graft	DD	developmental disability	FCE	functional capacity evaluation

Table-3-1, Continued

Abbreviations and Symbols

Abbreviation	Definition	Abbreviation	Definition	Abbreviation	Definition
FIM	Functional Independence Measure	Ⓘ	independent	MVA	motor vehicle accident
flex.	flexion	I&O	intake and output	N	Normal (muscle strength grade of 5)
fl oz	fluid ounce	IADL	instrumental activity of daily living	NA	not applicable, not available
FM	fine motor	ICU	intensive care unit		
FROM	functional range of motion	i.e.	that is	N/A	not applicable
ft.	foot, feet (the measurement, not the body part)	IEP	Individualized Education Program	NAD	no acute distress
		IM	intramuscular	NDT	neurodevelopmental treatment
F/U	follow-up	in.	inches	neg.	negative
FUO	fever of unknown origin	int.	internal	NG	nasogastric
		IP	inpatient, interphalangeal	NICU	neonatal intensive care unit
FWB	full weight bearing	IR	internal rotation	NKA	no known allergy
Fx	fracture	IV	intravenous	NKDA	no known drug allergy
G	Good (muscle strength grade of 4)	KAFO	knee-ankle-foot orthosis	NMES	neuromuscular electrical stimulation
GI	gastrointestinal	kg	kilogram	NOS	not otherwise specified
gm	gram	Ⓛ	left		
GSW	gunshot wound	lb.	pound	NPO	nothing by mouth
GYN	gynecology	LD	learning disability, learning disorder	NS	no show, not seen
h	hour	LE	lower extremity	NSAID	nonsteroidal anti-inflammatory drug
HA, H/A	headache	LLQ	left lower quadrant		
H&P	history and physical	LOC	loss of consciousness, level of consciousness	NSR	normal sinus rhythm
HBV	hepatitis B virus			NWB	nonweight bearing
HEENT	head, eyes, ears, nose, throat	LRTI	ligament reconstruction tendinous interposition	O	objective; oriented
HEP	home exercise program			O_2	oxygen
		LTG	long-term goal	OA	osteoarthritis
HHA	home health agency, home health aide	LUQ	left upper quadrant	OB	obstetrics
		m	murmur; meter; male	OBS	organic brain syndrome
HIPAA	Health Insurance Portability and Accountability Act	max	maximum	OCD	obsessive compulsive disorder
		MD	muscular dystrophy; medical doctor	OOB	out of bed
HIV	human immunodeficiency virus	meds.	medications	OP	outpatient
		MET	basal metabolic equivalent	OR	operating room
HOB	head of bed			ORIF	open reduction, internal fixation
HOH	hand over hand; hard of hearing	mg	milligram		
		MHz	megahertz	OT	occupational therapist, occupational therapy
HP	hot pack	MI	myocardial infarction	OTA	occupational therapy assistant
hr.	hour	min	minutes; minimum		
HR	heart rate	ml	milliliter	OTAS	occupational therapy assistant student
HRT	hormone replacement therapy	mm	millimeter		
		MMT	manual muscle test	OTC	over the counter
HS	bedtime	mo.	month	OTR	registered occupational therapist
Ht	height	mod	moderate		
HTN	hypertension	MP, MCP	metacarpophalangeal	OX4	oriented to time, place, person, situation
HVPC	high volt pulsed current	MRI	magnetic resonance imaging		
				oz	ounce
Hx	history	MS	multiple sclerosis	p̄	after

Table-3-1, Continued

Abbreviations and Symbols

P	plan; posterior; pulse; Poor (muscle strength grade of 2)	qt.	quart	STG	short-term goal
		$\circledR$	right	STM	short-term memory
		R	respiration	suppos	suppository
PA	posterior anterior, physician's assistant	RA	rheumatoid arthritis	sup	supination
		RBC	red blood cell count	T	temperature; Trace (muscle strength grade of 1)
PADL	personal activity of daily living	R.D.	registered dietician		
		re:	regarding		
PAM	physical agent modality	rehab	rehabilitation	TB	tuberculosis
		reps	repetitions	TBI	traumatic brain injury
PDD	pervasive developmental disorder	resp	respiratory; respiration	TEDS	thrombo-embolic disease stockings
		RICE	rest, ice, compression, elevation	TENS	transcutaneous electrical nerve stimulation
PE	physical examination; physical education	R.Ph.	registered pharmacist	TFCC	triangular fibrocartilage complex
		RLQ	right lower quadrant		
per	by	R/O	rule out		
peri.	perineal	ROM	range of motion	ther ex	therapeutic exercise
PET	positron emission tomography	ROS	review of symptoms	THR	total hip replacement
		R.T.	respiratory therapist	TIA	transient ischemic attack
Ph.D.	doctor of philosophy	RTC	return to clinic		
PIP	proximal interphalangeal	RTO	return to office	TKR	total knee replacement
		RUQ	right upper quadrant	TM(J)	temporomandibular (joint)
p.m., PM	afternoon; evening	RSD	reflex sympathetic dystrophy		
PMH	past medical history			TNR	tonic neck reflex (also ATNR; STNR)
PNF	proprioceptive neuro-muscular facilitation	Rx	recipe; Latin *take thou prescription*		
				t.o.	telephone order
PNI	peripheral nerve injury	$\circledS$	supervision	TOS	thoracic outlet syndrome
PNS	peripheral nervous system	$\overline{s}$	without		
		S	subjective	TPR	temperature, pulse, & respiration
POMR	problem oriented medical record	SBA	stand by assistance		
		SCI	spinal cord injury	TTWB	toe touch weight bearing
pos.	positive	SH	social history		
post op	postoperative	SI	sensory integration	tx.	treatment; traction
PRE	progressive resistive exercise	SIDS	sudden infant death syndrome	UA	urinalysis
				UE	upper extremity
pre op	preoperative	Sig:	instruction to patient	UMN	upper motor neuron
PRN	as needed	SLE	systemic lupus erythematosus	URI	upper respiratory infection
pro	pronation				
PROM	passive range of motion	SLP	speech-language pathologist	US	ultrasound
				UTI	urinary tract infection
pt.	patient	SOC	start of care	VC	vital capacity
PT	physical therapy, physical therapist	SOAP	subjective, objective, assessment, plan	VD	venereal disease
				v.o.	verbal orders
P/T	part time	SOB	shortness of breath	vol.	volume
PTA	physical therapist assistant; prior to admission	SNF	skilled nursing facility	VS	vital signs
		S/P	status post	W	watt
		SSRI	selective serotonin reuptake inhibitor	WBC	white blood cell; white blood count
PTSD	post traumatic stress disorder	STAT	immediately	WBAT	weight bearing as tolerated
PWB	partial weight bearing	STD	sexually transmitted disease		
Px	physical examination			w/c	wheelchair

Table-3-1, Continued

Abbreviations and Symbols

WDWN	well developed; well nourished	*Symbols*		→	to; progressing forward; approaching
wk.	week	1°	primary	~	approximately
WFL	within functional limits	2°	secondary; secondary to	@	at
WNL	within normal limits	Δ	change	=	equals
wt	weight	x1, x2	of 1 person; of 2 people	+	plus; positive (also abbreviated pos.)
x or X	times		Example: "transferred to toilet c̄ min Ⓐ x2"	−	minus; negative (also abbreviated neg.)
y.o.	year old			#	number (#1); pounds
yr.	year	♂	male	%	percent
		♀	female	&	and
		>	greater than	°	degree
		<	less than	"	inches
		↓	down; downward; decrease	'	feet
		↑	up; upward; increase	/	per
		↔	to and from		

Worksheet 3-1
Using Abbreviations

Translate each sentence written with abbreviations into full English phrases or sentences.

1. Pt. ① BADL.

2. Client reports ↓ pain ⓡ shoulder p̄ HP.

3. Resident w/c ↔ EOB with SBA.

4. Client c/o pain in ⓡ MCP joint p̄ ~ 5 min PROM.

5. Client w/c → mat c̄ sliding board max Ⓐ x2.

6. Pt. O x 4.

7. Client has SOB c̄ PRE.

8. Pt. has ↓ STM and OCD which limit IADL.

9. Pt. min Ⓐ AMB bed → toilet 2° ↓ balance.

10. Child's FM WFL to don AFO.

Worksheet 3-2

Using Abbreviations—Additional Practice

Shorten these notes using only the standard abbreviations in this chapter.

1. Client requires minimal assistance to stand and pull up clothing with partial weight bearing status of right lower extremity.

2. Patient is able to feed herself independently with use of built-up utensils.

3. Client has intact sensation in both upper extremities but complains of minimal pain.

4. Client has fifty-five degrees of passive range of motion in the left index distal interphalangeal joint which is within functional limits.

5. While sitting on edge of bed, client is able to put on her socks with standby assistance, but requires moderate assistance with putting on and taking off left shoe.

6. Student is independent in wheelchair mobility and basic activities of daily living.

7. Patient requires moderate assistance of two people to transfer from wheelchair to toilet and from toilet to wheelchair.

8. Patient's toe touch weight bearing status limits her performance of instrumental activities of daily living.

Worksheet 3-3
Deciphering Doctors' Orders and Abbreviations

Translate the following abbreviations into full English phrases or sentences.

1. Dx s/p Ⓡ TKR 2° OA; WBAT
   OT 2x/wk. for BADL, IADL

2. X-ray + Ⓛ index finger MC Fx 2° GSW

3. 5 y.o. child has pain 2° bone CA Ⓛ LE

4. Dx Ⓡ DRUJ Fx c̄ ORIF
   OT 3x/wk. for PAMs PRN, P/AROM, ADL, CPM

5. 1° Dx PTSD, 2° Dx OCD

6. 1° Dx DJD Ⓡ hip, 2° Dx COPD & CHF

7. Dx CAD, TIA

Worksheet 3-4

Deciphering Doctors' Orders and Abbreviations—More Practice

Translate the following abbreviations into full English phrases or sentences.

1. Dx PDD-NOS, ADHD
    OT: ADL, SI, FM
    2 x/wk. X 12 wks.

2. EMG – Ⓡ CTS and - TOS

3. Dx: s/p Ⓛ THR, pt. NWB Ⓛ LE, OOB c̄ walker
    OT eval. and tx; ADL, Ⓑ UE PREs
    3x/wk. X 4/wks.

4. MRI + TBI, VS stable, BRP

5. CXR – TB but + URI, pt. has DOE and FUO

6. Dx PTSD, ETOH abuse, HBV

Worksheet 3-5

Additional Practice

Shorten these notes using only the standard abbreviations in this chapter.

1. The patient was seen bedside for instruction in basic activities of daily living. She was able to perform bed mobility exercises with moderate assistance, but needed maximum assistance to put on her lower extremity garments and moderate assistance to put on upper extremity garments. She was able to go from a supine position to a sitting position with minimum assistance and from a sitting position to a standing position with moderate assistance.

2. The resident came to the occupational therapy clinic via wheelchair escort. The resident was observed to lean to his left. The resident needed verbal cues and minimum assistance in positioning his body in the wheelchair to maintain midline orientation and symmetrical posture. The resident transferred from his wheelchair to the toilet with moderate assistance of one person to help him keep his balance using a standing pivot transfer. He needed verbal cues and visual feedback from a mirror to maintain upright posture.

3. The patient was seen in the occupational therapy clinic for left distal radioulnar joint fracture. Patient is now ten weeks status post fracture. Patient also has an upper respiratory infection. He was seen for assessment of selected, relevant client factors. The left upper extremity shoulder flexion was a grade of 4, shoulder extension was a grade of 4, elbow flexion was a grade of 4, elbow extension was a grade of 4, wrist extension was a grade of 3 minus, wrist flexion was a grade of 3 minus, and grip strength was 8 pounds. The left upper extremity light touch is intact. The right upper extremity muscle grades and sensation are within functional limits.

Chapter 4

Avoiding Common Documentation Mistakes

Throughout your career as an OTA, you will encounter many opportunities to use your professional documentation skills. Of course, one essential responsibility of the OTA is to write in the health record. In addition, you will be writing notes and memos to colleagues and staff. You might even be involved with composing letters, reports, or marketing materials to send to insurance companies or other healthcare professionals. Your written and verbal communication is a reflection of you, the occupational therapy practitioner. It also reflects on your department and the profession of occupational therapy as a whole. Think about what someone will infer about you from documentation that has numerous errors in spelling and grammar. Perhaps people will question your credibility, your credentials, competence, or even your intelligence. They may have less respect for you or consider you to be careless, sloppy, or unprofessional. On the other hand, documentation that is well written, grammatically correct, well organized, and neat demonstrates professionalism and pride in your work.

Make use of readily available resources such as a dictionary, thesaurus, computer program or portable electronic devices to assist you with spelling and grammar as needed. Also, take the necessary time to write carefully and proofread your work. Rushing to complete documentation quickly can often result in sloppy, careless errors and inaccuracies in copying or recording information. This could possibly lead to serious consequences for you or the client. The following sections and worksheets will help you learn to avoid some common documentation mistakes.

Quotes and Paraphrasing

There are several ways to document what your client or another person has said. You can quote, or state what the person said exactly word for word, or you can paraphrase or summarize it. When quoting someone exactly, the person's specific words are used between a set of quotation marks. Remember that the punctuation to end the sentence stays within the quotation marks. If you are referring to the client's statement in the first person (I), the use of the letter I should be within the quotation marks. For example, to use a first person quote, you might write:

> *The client stated, "I will never be able to go back to work."*

If you, the therapist, are referring to the client in the third person (he, she), that pronoun would be outside of the quotation marks and you will just quote the exact words said. For example:

> *The client stated that he "will never be able to go back to work."*

If you are just paraphrasing or summarizing what another person said, you do not have to use quotation marks. Also, remember that an indirect question does not require a question mark. Here is an example of paraphrasing:

The client expressed doubts about returning to work.

Sometimes, you might just want to quote or emphasize a significant word or phrase. For example:

The client stated that he "will never" be able to return to his job.

Now look at some examples of how to record the same information in different ways:

Correct:

Patient stated, "I didn't sleep well last night."

Patient stated that he "didn't sleep well last night."

Patient stated that last night he didn't sleep well.

Patient stated that he slept poorly last night.

Incorrect:

Patient stated, "he didn't sleep well last night."

Patient stated, he "didn't sleep well last night."

Correct:

Mary stated she has "an ache" in her right hip.

Mary stated, "I have an ache in my right hip."

Incorrect:

Mary stated, "I have an ache in her right hip."

Mary stated "she has an ache in her right hip."

Correct:

The client asked, "Will I be able to walk soon?"

The client inquired if she would soon be able to ambulate.

The client asked if she would "be able to walk soon."

Incorrect:

The client asked "if she would be able to walk soon."

The client asked if she would "be able to walk soon?"

Worksheet 4-1
Quoting and Paraphrasing

In the following statements, determine which are correct (C) or incorrect (I). Pay close attention to punctuation.

1. _____ The child stated that she was extremely hungry.
2. _____ The child stated that "she was starving."
3. _____ The child "stated I am starving."
4. _____ The child indicated that she was "starving."
5. _____ The child stated "I am starving."

6. _____ The patient asked how to put her splint on?
7. _____ The patient asked "How do I put my splint on"?
8. _____ The patient asked about the proper way to put on her splint.
9. _____ The patient asked, "How do I put my splint on?"
10. _____ The patient asked "how to put her splint on."

11. _____ The client requested a new buttonhook.
12. _____ The client asked if "she could have a new buttonhook."
13. _____ The client asked, "Can I have a new buttonhook"?
14. _____ The client asked for a new buttonhook.
15. _____ The client asked, "Can I have a new buttonhook?"

16. _____ The client stated "he felt dizzy" as he stood at the kitchen counter.
17. _____ The client reported feeling "dizzy" while standing at the kitchen counter.
18. _____ While standing at the kitchen counter, the client stated "he felt dizzy."
19. _____ The client, while standing at the kitchen counter, stated I feel "dizzy."
20. _____ The client reported dizziness while standing at the kitchen counter.

Mini-Worksheet 4-2: Spelling

Students frequently misspell some common words used in OT documentation. For each of the pairs below, place a check mark next to the word that is spelled correctly.

1. __ defered   __ deferred   7. __ recieve   __ receive

2. __ definately   __ definitely   8. __ judgment   __ judgement

3. __ dining   __ dinning   9. __ rotator cup   __ rotator cuff

4. __ excercise   __ exercise   10. __ tolorate   __ tolerate

5. __ parrafin   __ paraffin   11. __ therapy puddy   __ therapy putty

6. __ transfering   __ transferring   12. __ independent   __ independant

Worksheet 4-3
Using Words Correctly

Students often misuse certain words that sound similar. Complete the following sentences by choosing the correct word from the two choices provided in parentheses.

1. The home health _____ gave the patient a shower. (aid or aide)

2. The client refused to _____ the doctor's diagnosis. (accept or except)

3. The traumatic brain injury will have a tremendous _____ on activities of daily living. (affect or effect)

4. If the client falls, she probably will _____ her hip due to osteoporosis. (brake or break)

5. The patient became short of _____ after ambulating to the bathroom. (breath or breathe)

6. The client stated she wanted to _____ ten pounds. (lose or loose)

7. The patient injured her _____ right hand which prevented her from writing. (dominant or dominate)

8. The occupational therapy room is _____ down the hallway than the physical therapy room. (farther or further)

9. The _____ caseload consists of 10 clients, as compared to 15 clients last week. (currant or current)

10. The OTR asked the patient to _____ the scissors down on the table. (lay or lie)

11. The weight of the pan was more _____ the patient could manage. (than or then)

12. The clients in the craft group put _____ projects away in the closet. (their or there)

13. The child was able to remain quiet and _____ while standing in line. (stationary or stationery)

14. The _____ of the school attended the IEP meeting. (principal or principle)

Capitals

When in doubt regarding use of capitals, always refer to a medical or college dictionary. Some of the more commonly confused situations regarding capitals are listed below and, according to the *Merriam-Webster's Guide to Punctuation and Style* (Merriam-Webster, 2001), the following rules pertain:

Capitalized	Example	Not capitalized	Example
Proper names in medical terminology	Parkinson disease, Babinski sign, Heimlich maneuver	Common nouns in medical terminology	measles, virus, flu, hysterectomy, biceps
Trade names of products and medications	Pampers diapers, Advil, Jobst glove	Generic drugs and products	disposable diapers, compression glove, aspirin
Specific organizations	American Occupational Therapy Association	Generic organizations	a book club, the church group
Academic degrees and professional designations after the person's name	Marie Morreale, OTR, CHT	General degrees or generic professional designations	an associate's degree, an occupational therapist
Exact test titles	Canadian Occupational Performance Measure	Generic tests	range of motion evaluation, a cognitive test
Specific department proper names	Healthy Hospital Occupational Therapy Department	Generic department names	an occupational therapy department, rehab department
Official titles as part of a name	Dr. Jones, Reverend Smith	Generic or descriptive titles	the doctor's office, the clergyman

Mini-Worksheet 4-4: Capitals

Underline the words that do not correctly follow the rules for capitals.

1. The OTA put the chart on the Physical Therapist's desk.

2. The Patient was going to see his Doctor this afternoon.

3. The OT Aide used velcro and Scotch Tape to fix Mrs. Smith's lapboard during the occupational therapy session.

4. The Doctor spoke to the child who has Chicken Pox.

5. The OTA Student performed a Manual Muscle Test on the client.

6. The client took Tylenol and Antacids before his Rotary Club Meeting.

Verb Tenses

Choose and use one verb tense within a paragraph. Consider the following:

*The OTA **has helped** Joe's fine motor skills; the PT **helped** Joe's balance. The special educator **had worked** with Joe so he could learn the school routine. The classroom aide **works** very closely with him every day.*

The above paragraph uses four different verb tenses: present perfect, past, past perfect, and present. Instead, it is better to choose and use only one verb tense.

Pronouns

Be careful to make the pronoun reference clear. If you say, *Jane and Mary agree that her skills are improving,* it is not clear if the "her" refers to Jane or refers to Mary. It is better to say *Jane and Mary agree that Mary's skills are improving.* Another incorrect example is *The OT's student put his goniometer in his lab coat pocket,* as it is not clear whose goniometer or whose pocket is being referred to. It would be better to say, *The OT student put the OT's goniometer in the OT's lab coat pocket.*

Another common student error is using pronouns that don't agree with the subject to which they refer. For example, it is incorrect to write *One person in the group wasn't able to complete their craft project.* Instead, it should read, *One person in the group wasn't able to complete his craft project* (or her craft project if referring to a female).

You must also determine if the subject and pronoun are singular or plural for consistency. Another incorrect statement would be *They will hurt themself if they lift too much weight.* The correct version should be *They will hurt themselves if they lift too much weight.*

Plurals and Possessives

The proper way to indicate plurals or possessives can sometimes seem confusing. We will now look at several situations that students sometimes have difficulty with. According to the *Publication Manual of the American Psychological Association* (American Psychological Association [APA], 2001), to indicate the plural of an abbreviation, usually just the letter "s" is added. For example:

The OTs each supervised two OTAs.

The MDs wanted to use the conference room.

Remember that when you are showing that something belongs to one person or object (singular possessive), most of the time you use an apostrophe before the letter "s". Here are some examples:

The client's right hand was minimally edematous.

That chair's armrests are broken.

The OTA's goniometer was in her desk.

When you have more than one person or object and want to indicate that something belongs to all of them (plural possessive), the apostrophe goes after the letter "s." For example:

The clients' charts were in the file cabinet.

The OTA students' lunches were free in the hospital cafeteria.

The occupational therapy assistants' treatment notes were cosigned by their supervisors.

The OTAs' patients were all in the waiting room.

Mini-Worksheet 4-5: Pronouns, Plurals, Possessives

Look at the following sentences and determine the incorrect components in each sentence.

1. The three client's appointments were all canceled today because their OTA was ill.
2. The OTAs lab coat was new.
3. The OTA students resumé was reviewed by the OT.
4. The childs parent's both attended the therapy session.
5. The children almost hurt theirselves when they collided with each other in the hallway.
6. The nurses patient gave them all flowers.
7. The PT's and OT's had the day off.
8. The occupational therapists' paperwork was on her desk.
9. One of the client's lost their splint.

Now you are ready to begin writing SOAP notes. Always remember that your documentation is a reflection of you as both an individual and occupational therapy professional. Make a concerted effort to use correct spelling, punctuation, and grammar in all your professional writing. When in doubt, refer to a dictionary, spell checker, or style manual to assure accuracy. The rest of this manual will take you step by step through the process of writing SOAP notes and help you to develop clinical reasoning skills. You will be soon be thinking and writing like an OTA.

From Borcherding S, Morreale M. *The OTA's Guide to Writing SOAP Notes, Second Edition.* © 2007 SLACK Incorporated.

Chapter 5

Writing the "S"—Subjective

The first section of the SOAP note contains **SUBJECTIVE** information obtained from the client. This "S" section expresses the client's perspective regarding the client's condition or treatment. Subjective data is information that cannot necessarily be verified or measured during the treatment session. In this section, the occupational therapy practitioner records the client's report of limitations, concerns, and problems, as well as what the client communicated that was relevant to treatment. This can include statements regarding significant complaints of pain, fatigue, or expressions of feelings, attitudes, concerns, goals, and plans. Appropriate, direct quotes are often used in the subjective section of the SOAP note. In this case, it is understood that the statement comes from the individual receiving the therapy, unless otherwise stated. This subjective information will have more significance and relevance to the rest of your note if it specifically pinpoints an issue rather than just noting a vague or general comment from the client. For instance, if the client tells you, "My hand hurts," you may probe further, asking "Where does it hurt?" or "When does it hurt?" or "Describe what it feels like." This will allow your note to communicate more detailed information on the individual's condition by recording the client's own description or perception: *Client states he has sharp pain in his Ⓡ hand when he tries to lift a heavy pan or grocery bag.* You may quote, paraphrase, or summarize what the client said. Review Chapter 4 for specific information regarding the use of proper grammar and punctuation for direct and indirect quotes.

Examples of "S" Statements

- "I don't need therapy."

- Resident reports pain in Ⓡ hand when using computer keyboard.

- Patient expressed doubts about ever getting better and then began to cry.

- Client reports, "I keep blowing up at home, and yelling at everyone, and I don't know what to do about it."

- "I can't tie my shoes or zip my coat."

- Veteran reports that his fingers "look kind of dead."

- Client reports that stress and anxiety keep her awake at night.

- Child reports that she is too embarrassed to wear her leg brace and splints because the other students make fun of her.

- Patient expresses a desire to return to her factory job as soon as possible. She states that she needs to be able to lift 20 lbs., stand for 3 hour periods, and put together small parts with screws and twist ties. She is also concerned about the financial implications of her inability to work 2° her injury.

- Consumer reports being fearful of leaving her home.

- Client reports that his doctor has ordered "some home care for a few days to work on transfers."

- Client reported that her hands "always feel better after the paraffin treatments." She also stated, "My short-term goal is to be able to use the computer, and my long-term goal is to return to work."

- Client called the emergency line last night to report a burning sensation in her "gut", which made her afraid she was going to die. Today she reports that she has been worrying about dying and has not showered since the day before yesterday.

- Resident stated that she has experienced several episodes of bladder incontinence when trying to make it to the bathroom.

- Client stated, "I feel so stressed out about losing my job that I can't concentrate or sleep. I don't feel like myself anymore." She also reported that exercise, gardening, and volunteer work are her primary coping strategies, and that she would like to learn more about relaxation techniques.

- Student stated that she would like to be able to perform toilet hygiene Ⓘ at school.

- Patient reports "pins and needles" in the dorsal Ⓛ forearm.

Sometimes the client is not able to speak or does not make any relevant comments. In such cases, include that information in the "S" section. For example:

- Client unable to communicate due to aphasia.

- Client did not speak without cueing.

- Patient communicated using his message board that he wants to be able to walk again.

- Resident does not clearly verbalize during treatment, but smiles and nods appropriately when asked questions.

In certain instances, the "S" part of the SOAP note might reflect an important statement, problem, or concern that the client's caregiver or family communicates to the clinician regarding the client. Also, when treating infants and very young children, you may report what the parent says. For example:

- Mother reports child was able to sit unsupported for 45 seconds yesterday.

- Caregiver reports client refuses to wear her splint.

- Husband reports, "I am really concerned that she is going to kill herself."

- Parent reports infant has an ear infection and is "very cranky today."

- Daughter reports pt. lives with her and sometimes forgets to turn off the stove. Daughter states she works full-time. She is concerned that her mother is alone and unsupervised during the day and could "hurt herself or burn down the house."

Except for infants, people who are unable to communicate, and special circumstances, the "S" section is usually reserved for the client's view. If a client is deaf or only speaks a different language, it is important to have someone present who can interpret or translate all communication between the client and clinician. This should also be recorded in the note.

Common Errors

Not Using Communication Time With the Client Effectively

The most common error that new OTAs make in gathering subjective information is in failing to make good use of communication with the client during treatment sessions. It is important to make the client feel comfortable and at ease. However, rather than using most of the therapy time to talk socially, a good OTA will use the time to listen effectively and to ask questions that will elicit pertinent information about the client's attitudes and concerns. This information can then be used to ensure effective treatment as well as appropriate documentation. Instead of discussing the weather or Monday Night Football, why not ask your client how he thinks he is doing in therapy or what his feelings are related to his upcoming discharge placement? As OTAs gain experience, they begin to use the treatment session to obtain relevant data regarding such things as occupational history, functional status, prior level of functioning, priorities, motivation, and family support. Effective communication and interviewing during intervention sessions can seem just like a conversation on the surface. But, as a skilled OTA, you are carefully directing the conversation to topics that are meaningful to client care rather than allowing it to remain superficial. Use this opportunity to expand the client's occupational profile and gather data that is vital to providing the very best occupational therapy possible. When conversing with your client, guide the discussion to your client's history, problems, needs, concerns, strengths, support systems, living situation, and goals for treatment. Without knowing these things from your client's point of view, you will have difficulty planning effective treatment. When an OTA does not listen effectively during treatment, the "S" may read:
- Client talked about grandchildren visiting.
  -OR-
- Patient said "ouch" when elbow was ranged beyond 45°.
  -OR-
- Resident stated that her lunch tasted very good.

While these statements are within the scope of the "S," they are not particularly helpful pieces of information to spend time and space reporting.

Not Writing Concise, Coherent Statements

The second most common error new OTAs make when writing the subjective section of the note is that of simply listing any remarks the client makes about his condition.

For example, during one treatment session the client said the following:

"I'm wobbly as I get out today."

"I can't feel anything with my hands."

Client expressed dizziness after bending down to touch the floor while in a seated position. Client acknowledged improvement in his sitting balance in comparison to the previous week.

These statements generally involve stability, balance, and safety issues. While the quotations are a very objective way of reporting information, and all the remarks are relevant to the intervention session, it is more effective to summarize the client's statements more concisely and coherently. Rather than listing each of these statements separately in the "S" section of the note, organize and record them in a more professional manner. For example:

Client expressed lack of sensation in both hands and dizziness in sitting position with dynamic movement (a "wobbly" sensation). He also acknowledged improvement in sitting balance since last week.

-OR-

Client acknowledged improved sitting balance compared to previous week. However, he expressed dizziness after bending down while sitting, and reported feeling "wobbly." Client also reported inability to feel anything with his hands.

In the next two exercises, you will have the opportunity to select coherent and concise "S" statements.

Worksheet 5-1
Choosing a Subjective Statement

A female client is recovering after a Ⓛ CVA. This observation note was written after one of her occupational therapy treatment sessions.

O: Client seen in rehab clinic for 30 minutes for UE activities to ↑ AROM in Ⓡ shoulder, activity tolerance, UE strength, and dynamic standing balance, in order to ↑ independence in ADL tasks.

BADL: Client seen in room for instruction in safety techniques and adaptive equipment use in toileting. Client required use of bilateral grab bars in bathroom to sit ↔ stand safely. Client first attempted to stand while pulling on walker and one grab bar. Client was instructed on safety issues and the use of bilateral grab bars, which she reported understanding.

Performance skills: Client sit → stand CGA for balance. Client worked on activity tolerance, dynamic standing balance, and ↑ AROM in Ⓡ shoulder by moving canned goods from counter to cupboard for 5 minutes before needing to sit and rest 2 minutes. She then participated in activities to ↑ dynamic standing balance by pouring liquid from a pitcher while standing CGA for balance. After a 1-minute rest, client continued activities to ↑ dynamic standing balance and safety in ADL activities by pushing wheeled walker while picking up objects from floor c̄ a reacher.

Client factors: AROM in right shoulder abduction < 90°. PROM Ⓡ shoulder abduction WNL.

The treatment session included all of the following. Which would be best to use as the subjective section of the SOAP note?

1. Client remarked that her grandson will be coming to visit later in the week, and that she will be very glad to see him.

2. Client was cooperative and engaged in social conversation throughout the treatment session.

3. Client reports that she feels "pretty good" today.

4. Client says she has difficulty moving Ⓡ UE, although she does not know why it will not move. She reports, "It really doesn't hurt. It's just tight."

5. Nursing staff report client is unsafe to toilet self independently.

Worksheet 5-2
Writing Concise, Coherent Statements

Your client is recovering from a Ⓛ total hip replacement. During an occupational therapy treatment session, the client makes the following statements.

- "I used that dressing stick and sock aid like you showed me to get dressed without bending down this morning.
- It's getting easier for me to get dressed now.
- My hip doesn't hurt when I stand up or sit down; especially with that new toilet seat you got for me.
- My daughter said they delivered all that bathroom equipment to her house yesterday."

Using these statements, write your own concise and organized version for the "S" portion of the SOAP note.

S:

Chapter 6

Writing the "O"—Objective

The second part of the note is the **OBJECTIVE** section. This is where you will record all measurable, quantifiable, and observable data obtained during your client's occupational therapy treatment session. In this section, you present a picture or synopsis of the entire intervention session. Once you begin looking at things with your professional eyes, they can look and seem quite different. Instead of simply seeing a child playing with a toy, you now begin to make skilled observations such as noting the child's asymmetrical posture, his hand preference, balance, ability to cross midline, and his pinch and grasp patterns. A student or novice clinician may have difficulty figuring out what kind of material to include and what to omit in the "O" section. At first, your "O" may tend to be longer than that of an experienced OTA, but with time you will learn to write notes that are both complete and concise.

Organization of the "O"

There are different ways to organize the information gleaned from your observations. One way is to present the information chronologically, discussing each treatment event in the order it occurred during that treatment session.

> *Resident seen bedside for 45 minutes for skilled BADL instruction. Once set up, resident was able to wash face and upper body with min Ⓐ and use of a wash mitt while sitting on EOB. Client also was instructed in use of long-handled hairbrush and electric toothbrush. She demonstrated ability to use these items to perform grooming tasks with min Ⓐ and two 60-second rest periods. Resident then applied make-up with set up and min Ⓐ while sitting up in bed. She expressed satisfaction regarding being finally able to participate in a "normal morning routine."*

Alternately, you may choose to organize your information into categories. When categorizing your information, choose the categories that make the most sense for your note. For example, suppose that today you saw a home care client for a cooking session in her kitchen. She needs to be able to prepare a light meal independently once her home health aide is discontinued. You don't know her level of safety awareness or her ability to perform all steps of the activities while using a walker. You wonder if her strength and activity tolerance are adequate for cooking, and you also want to assess her judgment, problem solving, and ability to adhere to THR precautions. You choose the following categories:

- Functional mobility
- UE Range and strength
- Activity tolerance
- Cognition

Your note might look like this:

O: Client seen at home for 1 hour for skilled instruction in compensatory techniques for cooking.

Functional mobility: Client used walker to maneuver throughout kitchen with min verbal cues to place walker in appropriate position for reaching objects in kitchen. Client was instructed in use of walker basket and wheeled cart to transport items.

UE ROM and strength: WFL for reaching items in drawers and upper cabinets and putting dishes in the sink Ⓘ. UE strength adequate for opening refrigerator door, using manual can opener, and pouring soup in and out of small pot. Client required min Ⓐ to use reacher to obtain item from bottom shelf in refrigerator.

Activity tolerance: Client able to stand for 10 minutes to heat soup at stove and make sandwich at counter. Client then required a 3-minute break. Client then able to stand at sink for 5 minutes to wash dishes.

Cognitive: Client able to respond to verbal instructions and questions with correct response 3/3 times. Client said she did not think it would be safe for her to use the oven at this time and would use the toaster oven instead. Client able to problem solve and safely adhere to all THR precautions.

There is no list of "correct" categories. You must use your clinical judgment to determine what is appropriate to include, summarize, or categorize. If the client has no deficits in a particular area, it is not necessary to address that category in the note. In choosing categories, you could use the *Framework* categories (AOTA, 2002), as these are useful in any practice setting.

- Areas of occupation
- Performance skills
- Performance patterns
- Client factors
- Activity demands
- Context

In some instances, the *Framework* categories may be too broad for your purposes. You might choose categories that relate more specifically to your client and your practice setting. You may want to consider some of the following:

- Basic and instrumental ADL task performance: Note how each of the performance skills and client factors observed impact completion of ADL tasks. Include assist levels and required set-up, any adaptive equipment, compensatory techniques, and methods used. Also include extent and type of cuing and response, family/caregiver education, positioning, and client's response to the intervention provided.
- Work and prevocational task performance: Note activity demands for work, ability to perform job tasks, consider career and transitional planning, and development of vocational skills.
- Leisure and play: Consider physical, cognitive, psychosocial, and developmental factors regarding participation in leisure activities, note barriers to play and leisure, skill development, and appropriateness of leisure time and choices.

- Posture and balance: Note whether balance was static or dynamic for sitting and standing. Consider whether the client leans in one direction, has rotated posture, even or uneven weight distribution. Notice position of the head, upper extremities, trunk, and symmetry. Note what feedback or cues were needed to maintain or restore balance.
- Coordination and dexterity: Note if dominant hand is affected, type of prehension patterns used, ability to grasp and maintain grasp of objects without dropping, reach and purposeful release, proximal control, precision handling, in-hand manipulation, gross vs. fine motor ability. Consider ability to manage bimanual tasks.
- Swelling or edema: Give girth or volumetric measurements if possible, pitting or nonpitting, including levels if pitting.
- Pain: Describe or qualify the pain and note the frequency and location. Consider how pain impacts the areas of occupation and performance patterns.
- Muscle, bone, and joint functions: Consider if PROM, AROM, strength, and structural alignment are adequate for performing occupational tasks.
- Movement patterns in affected upper extremity: Note motor planning, tone, tremors, synergy pattern, facilitation required, stabilization, body movement, substitution, or compensatory motions.
- Ability to follow instructions: Note attention, behavior, type and amount of instruction required, such as physical, verbal or visual cuing, ability to follow one-, two-, or three-step directions.
- Cognitive status: Report on task initiation, verbal responses, approach to the task, ability to stay on task, sequencing, oriented X 4 (identifying time, place, person, and situation), requirements for cuing, number of steps successfully completed in task, judgment (recognition of impairments, impulsivity, safety), ability to respond to written or verbal directions.
- Neurological factors: Note sensory losses (specific), perseveration (motor, speech), motor deficit, praxis, damage to innervations (spasticity, synergy, flaccidity, rigidity), unilateral neglect, bilateral integration, tremors.
- Functional mobility: Note the kind of assistance, cues, adaptive techniques, special devices or equipment required for the client to reposition self in bed, walk, propel a wheelchair, and use public transportation or drive.
- Activity tolerance: Note level of energy and endurance during tasks and impact on occupational performance.
- Psychosocial factors: Note client's overall mood, affect, ability to interact with others, and appropriateness of behavior. Also note family support, coping mechanisms, response to changes in body image, ability to adapt and make realistic discharge decisions for self.

Additional Categories for Mental Health or Behavioral Medicine (Mason, personal communication, 2001)

- Social interaction: Note awareness of others in the group, length of conversations, initiation of conversation, interaction with peers or leader in a group setting.
- Judgment and problem solving: Include any impulsivity, safety awareness, ability to identify and correct errors. Consider ability to make appropriate decisions.
- Behavior: Report on agitation, anxiety, lethargy, affect, compulsivity, demanding behavior.
- Appearance: Note grooming, hygiene, choice of appropriate attire.
- Work skills: Include promptness, time management, concentration, attention span, ability to follow direction, organization of task, including preparation and clean up.

Four Steps to Writing Good Observations

Step 1: Begin With a Statement About the Setting and Purpose of the Activity

If you are working directly on **occupation based tasks**, use the following format for your opening sentence:

Client seen for _____ minutes _____ for _____
(In what setting)   (Purpose of the treatment session)

Some facilities require that you document the number of minutes for the total session or for each specific occupational therapy service the client receives. This is usually for billing purposes such as the use of CPT codes. Your documentation is the basis for answering any questions that might arise regarding the amount or specific type of occupational therapy treatment the patient received. Facilities that do not charge for occupational therapy by the number of minutes may not require that you document the length of time a client was seen. However, you do still need to document the skilled services that were provided.

If the session is centered on improving **client factors** such as active range of motion, strengthening, activity tolerance, or dynamic balance, then add a reference to **the relevant area of occupation** in the opening line:

Client seen for _____ minutes _____ for _____
(In what setting)   (Purpose)
for _____
   (For what expected functional gain)

For example:

Pt. seen 30 minutes in OT craft group to improve interpersonal skills and promote leisure skills development.

Child seen for 45 minutes in clinic to increase selective attention and fine motor manipulation as a prerequisite to enhanced play and BADL tasks.

Client seen for 60 minutes in hospital room to provide skilled instruction in energy conservation in IADL activities and for explanation of client education materials on energy conservation.

Consumer participated in role-play activity for 30 minutes in assertion group in order to explore alternative ways to get his social needs met.

Resident seen for 20 minutes in room at sink for instruction in energy conservation and adaptive strategies for grooming Ⓘ.

Student seen in sensory integration playroom to address sensory defensiveness in classroom activities.

Pt. seen in OT clinic for 60 minutes for thermal modalities, P/AROM, and strengthening exercises Ⓡ UE in order to prepare for return to work.

Resident seen for ½ hour UE exercise group to ↑ strength for w/c mobility.

Showing Your Skill

It is important to show the need for your skill as an OTA in the very first sentence of your "O." For example, instead of saying "*Client seen for 45 minutes bedside for dressing,*" or "*Client seen for 45 minutes bedside for ADL training,*" you might say: "*Client seen for 45 minutes bedside for instruction in **compensatory dressing techniques**.*"

Here are some examples for other situations:

*Client seen for 30 minutes in OT kitchen for **instruction in time management techniques**.*

*Child and parents seen for 30 minutes in technology clinic for instruction in **use of assistive technology for classroom activities**.*

*Resident seen for 45 minutes bedside for instruction in **use of adaptive equipment to increase safety in ADL tasks**.*

*Consumer seen for 45 minutes bedside to **facilitate attention to** Ⓛ **side during self-care activities**.*

*Pt. seen 1 hour in OT clinic for **fabrication of** Ⓛ **cock-up splint to** ↓ **pain for ADL**.*

*Child seen for 45 minutes in classroom for **adaptation of backpack to facilitate** Ⓘ **use**.*

*Resident seen for 30 minutes in OT life skills group for **instruction in stress management techniques**.*

Step 2: Follow the Opening Sentence With a Summary of What You Observed

After the setting and purpose have been established, you will discuss the intervention you have just completed, either in chronological order or organized into categories. Some notes work best when reported chronologically, and others work better with categories.

Julie is a 27-year-old mother of 2 children ages 2 and 4. She is employed in a manufacturing job that involves lifting 30 lb. boxes. She is currently unable to work due to back pain from a herniated disc in her lumbar area. She complains of pain when doing her housework, and tells you that she wants to be able to perform IADL and work tasks without pain. As part of her occupational profile, the OTR delegates several tasks to the OTA that need to be observed and modified. You, the OTA, are asked to have this client demonstrate some IADL and work tasks. As you watch her take items from the refrigerator, wash the dishes, sweep and vacuum the floor, and lift a box from the floor to a chair, you find that her body mechanics are poor and that she would benefit from client education. If you reported on your session using chronological order, you might say:

O: Client seen for 30 minutes in OT clinic for assessment of low back pain and instruction in proper body mechanics. Client sits asymmetrically with weight shifted to her Ⓛ hip. Client demonstrated the way she usually removes items from the refrigerator, washes dishes, cleans the floors, and lifts. She was then instructed in proper body mechanics for completing these tasks, using a golfer's lift, squats, stepping toward the item she wishes to retrieve, facing the load and keeping it close to her body. Client demonstrated these techniques correctly and was given education materials to remind her of correct positioning.

If you wanted to put the same information into categories, you might say:

Client seen for 30 minutes in OT clinic for assessment of low back pain and instruction in proper body mechanics.

Bending and lifting: Client demonstrated her usual way of moving items from low surfaces to higher ones, demonstrating incorrect body mechanics in back extension and bending at the waist.   After instruction in using golfer's lift or squat, client demonstrated ability to use these techniques correctly in lifting and work activities after 2 attempts.

Transporting: Client exhibited torque in the spine in transporting items such as dishes. After instruction in sidestepping, facing the load and keeping it close to the body, client demonstrated proper use of these techniques with less reported pain.

Reaching: IADL tasks such as sweeping and vacuuming also habitually performed with rotation and overextension of the back. After instruction and demonstration of moving the body rather than overextending the arms, and keeping the load close to the body, client demonstrated correct body mechanics in performing reaching tasks with decreased pain.

Client education: Client given educational material to remind her of correct positioning for task and client reported that she understood what to do.

In this case, the chronological note works better because there is some repetition in the categorized version, and the categorized version is also longer. However, some notes are better if they are divided into sections. Categories help an inexperienced OTA to focus on the performance skills the client is demonstrating rather than the treatment media that is being used to facilitate these skills. It also helps other professionals to find pertinent information more quickly when they read your note. In the next exercise, you will review a chronological note that would work better in categories.

Worksheet 6-1
Organizing the "O" With Categories

Consider the following chronological observation:

Child seen for 60 minutes in daycare setting to work on reach/grasp/release and feeding skills. With min Ⓐ for facilitation of movement at elbow, child demonstrated ability to use Ⓛ UE to reach, grasp, and release 5 objects with 1 – 2 verbal cues per object and used Ⓡ UE to stabilize self for unsupported sitting at table. Child was able to feed self Ⓘ c̄ ~ 50% spillage, but demonstrated significant limitations in chewing action c̄ ~ 3 rotary chews & swallowing ~ 90% of food without chewing. Child required verbal cues throughout session to maintain attention to task. Child wore soft spica thumb splint for entire tx. session.

   How would you divide this information into categories to make it more organized and easier to read? Choose 3 to 4 categories and redistribute the information above into the categories you have chosen.

Step 3: Don't Duplicate Services

Make sure that your intervention is specific to occupational therapy as third party payers will not pay for duplication of services. While there will naturally be some overlap among rehabilitation disciplines, make sure you record what occupational therapy is doing differently. For example, physical therapy might be working with a client on ambulation with the goal of teaching use of an ambulation device or working on ambulation distance. Occupational therapy might work with this same client on using the ambulation device for a **specific functional activity**, such as safely loading the dishwasher or getting clothes out of a closet. If both occupational therapy and physical therapy are working on transfers, perhaps physical therapy is working on transfers to the mat or wheelchair and occupational therapy is working on transfers to the toilet or tub using adaptive equipment. If the speech therapist is working on reading a newspaper to facilitate articulation and language, the occupational therapy practitioner might be using the newspaper to facilitate cognitive skills and problem solving, such as locating classified ads or the movie schedule.

Step 4: Make Your Note Professional, Concise, and Specific

The "**O**" section does not need to be written in complete sentences but it does need to make sense. Give complete information in the most concise form possible. It is imperative that certain details be included. For example, ROM must be specified as passive, active, or assistive and must indicate the action and joint at which the movement occurred. UE or LE must indicate which UE or LE. Level of physical or verbal assistance must be specified if assistance was given.

When you are documenting test results, it is helpful to put them into a chart like the one below, rather than burying them in a narrative.

Sensory testing of Ⓛ hand revealed:
Hot/cold: intact
Sharp/dull: impaired over volar surface, intact over dorsal surface
Stereognosis: absent

Below are some examples of wording changes that make your wording more professional, concise, or specific.

Rather than saying: "Resident flopped down onto bed short of breath, closed her eyes and moaned. Resident laid in bed with min Ⓐ to position herself."
You might say: "Client observed to be fatigued following tx. session and required min Ⓐ for positioning in bed."

Rather than saying: "Veteran had to use a trapeze to sit up."
You might say: "Supine → sit using trapeze."

Rather than saying: "Client put the board in place to make a sliding board transfer."
You might say: "Client positioned sliding board for transfer."

When first learning to write client observations, it is hard to decide what to include and what to leave out. At first, it is best to include too much data, rather than take a chance on omitting something important. As your observational skills become more refined, it will become second nature to include all the important data, and the "**O**" section of your notes will begin to be more concise. Here is a client observation written by an inexperienced OTA. In an effort to include all the necessary data, this note is too "wordy".

Client was seen in therapy room for hot pack and Ⓡ UE strengthening. Client first had a hot pack applied to Ⓡ shoulder for 20 minutes. After the hot pack came off, client was asked to clasp hands together and raise arms above head 30X. Pt was then instructed to cross her midline and touch her opposite shoulder with Ⓡ UE. Client required 6 rest periods for completion. Client completed tasks Ⓘ. Client was then introduced to weight and pulley system. Client was asked to specify how much weight she thought she could do. She responded with 5#. Client did 30 reps of the pulley system with 5# in shoulder flexion to strengthen her rotator cuff to decrease the probability of dislocating her shoulder again.

An OTA with more experience might have written a more concise note:

Client treated in clinic for prevention of further Ⓡ shoulder dislocation. Hot pack applied to Ⓡ shoulder for 20 min followed by the following Ⓡ UE strengthening exercises for rotator cuff:
   Ⓑ clasped hand shoulder flexion and extension x 30 repetitions
   Horizontal adduction Ⓡ hand to Ⓛ shoulder x 30 repetitions
   Ⓡ shoulder flexion pulleys with 5# wt. x 30 repetitions

You will notice, however, that there is another problem with this note besides the fact that it is wordy. It also sounds like a physical therapy note rather than an occupational therapy note. This note needs to have functional components added, although they do not have to be in the "**O**." A statement from the client in the "**S**" about what she is unable to do with an injured rotator cuff and a statement in the "**A**" and/or "**P**" indicating functional problems/goals would suffice to make it a good occupational therapy note. Notice that being more concise means knowing what information can be omitted without compromising the quality of the observation.

It is possible to be **too** concise, omitting necessary information. For example, consider the following "**O**" from an inpatient occupational therapy session.

O: Client seen bedside for instruction in dressing techniques.

This "**O**" does not provide much information. When additional information is added, we learn quite a bit more about the session with this client:

O: Client seen bedside for skilled instruction in dressing techniques. Client exhibited some difficulty with sequencing and attempted to don slacks before underwear. Client also required min verbal cues to attend to Ⓛ side to place Ⓛ arm in shirt sleeve. Fine motor skills were WFL to manage buttons but moderate Ⓐ required to line up and fasten buttons properly 2° inattention to detail.

It is a matter of carefully balancing the need to be complete when writing the "**O**" with the need to be concise. In the next exercise, you will have an opportunity to make an observation more concise, without losing any of its informational content.

Worksheet 6-2
Being More Concise

Revise the following treatment observations to make the note complete but more concise:

O: Pt seen bedside for BADL. Client ambulated ~36 inches to shower stall with SBA for safety. Client instructed to complete shower while sitting. Client performed shower with SBA to manage IV line. Client able to wash upper and lower body ① and dry entire body after completing shower. Client required ~20 minutes to complete shower. Client then ambulated ~36 inches to chair and sat. Client needed verbal cues to remain seated while donning underwear and pants. Client able to dress upper body ① and lower body p̄ verbal cues for sitting. Client demonstrated good sitting balance, but needed SBA for standing balance. Following shower, client stated he would like to take a nap and was assisted back into bed.

This chapter has explained the basic components for writing the objective part of your SOAP note. The "O" section needs to be organized, concise, and must summarize what skilled OT services were provided in what setting. However, to make your documentation even better, there are other factors to consider when writing the "O" part of an occupational therapy note. The next chapter will provide you with additional tips for making your notes appear more accurate, professional, and complete. Remember, as you practice and gain clinical experience, your documentation skills will become much easier.

Chapter 7

Tips for Writing a Better "O"

This chapter contains additional tips to refine and improve your documentation skills. By incorporating these principles, your notes will appear more professional and complete, and you will be more likely to comply with third party payer guidelines.

Focus on Function

Make certain that occupation is integral to the note. In an intervention session devoted to self-care activities, function is obvious. In other circumstances, function must be addressed separately in order to justify skilled occupational therapy. Sessions where modalities are used or sessions devoted to treating client factors such as strength, range of motion, and endurance all need function emphasized in the treatment note. For example, although the note below is an observation of a session that was devoted to client factors, it contains a statement about the functional intent of the exercises.

> *O: Client seen bedside for AROM and strengthening of Ⓛ UE **in order to regain ability to dress self**. Client performed self-ranging exercises sitting on EOB c̄ standby Ⓐ for balance and verbal instructions to correct errors. Client was verbally cued X5 to reach higher with Ⓛ UE during shoulder flexion AROM.*

Document Use of Physical Agent Modalities Properly

OTs and OTAs often use physical agent modalities (PAMs) as a means to improve client factors such as decreasing pain and edema, increasing passive and active ROM and promoting wound healing. However, according to AOTA (2003b), the sole use of a PAM is not considered to be occupational therapy unless it is linked to occupational performance. Therefore, it is important to document **how the PAM will enable the client to perform specific functional tasks**. In addition, since another OT or OTA might be treating the client in your absence, it is necessary to document the proper parameters for the modality to ensure accuracy, safety, and consistent follow through. Always remember it is essential that occupational therapy practitioners who administer PAMs have service competency, follow ethical guidelines, and always adhere to state laws and regulations (AOTA, 2003b). Use Table 7-1 as a guide when documenting the use of PAMs.

Table 7-1.

PAM Checklist for Documentation

Part and Place where modality is applied on the body (e.g., right shoulder, left dorsal wrist)

Parameters (time, temperature, intensity, etc.)

Positioning considerations (limb placed in stretched position, digits wrapped in flexion, active exercise while modality applied, etc.)

Purpose/Preparation for what functional or therapeutic task or goal (e.g., pain relief, PROM/ stretching, ADL, scar management). Relate to occupational performance.

Patient response/Problems (tolerance, modifications required, other pertinent issues)

Here are some examples for recording use of PAMs:

Hot pack applied 20 minutes to ℝ wrist to ↓ pain and ↑ AROM to enable performance of kitchen tasks (e.g., lifting pots, cutting vegetables). Wrist placed in flexed position for stretch and client's skin checked at 5 and 10 minutes and upon removal of hot pack. No problems noted and client reports wrist "feels much looser after heat." Client then was instructed in use of an ergonomic knife to chop vegetables and demonstrated ability to lift a small pan containing 2 cups water without report of pain.

US applied to reduce pain and ↑ ROM Ⓛ shoulder to enable return to work. Pt. supine while continuous US applied 5 minutes to Ⓛ shoulder at 1MHz and 1 W/cm². Pt. tolerated US well and then worked on job simulation task of stacking 1 and 2 lb. cans on shelves c̄ Ⓛ UE. Pt. now able to flex Ⓛ shoulder 158° and stack 30 cans without report of pain. Pt. also able to lift and carry 10 lb. grocery bag 40 feet.

Fluidotherapy 110° for 15 minutes to Ⓛ wrist and hand. Client performed AROM wrist and hand during fluidotherapy tx. to increase grasp and release for precision tool handling. Wrist flexion ↑ 15° and index MCP ↑ 18° p̄ fluidotherapy.

Write From the Client's Point of View and Avoid Mentioning Yourself

The focus of good professional writing should be on the client and not the clinician (Kettenbach, 2004). Turn your sentences around so that the client is the subject of your sentence.

Rather than saying:	"The OTA put the client's shoes on for him."
You might say:	"Client Ⓓ in donning shoes."
Rather than saying:	"OTA instructed the client and family in energy conservation techniques."
You might say:	"Client and family were instructed in energy conservation techniques and demonstrated understanding by performing correctly."

Focus on the *Client's Response* to the Intervention Provided, Rather Than on What the OTA Did

Rather than saying: "Client was reminded about hip precautions."
You might say: "Attempting to don shoes, client required 3 verbal cues to keep hip in correct alignment."

Rather than saying: "Client was asked orientation questions pertaining to the time of day."
You might say: "When verbally cued to look at watch, client was unable to correctly identify time."

Rather than saying: "Client reminded to relax when interacting with sales clerk."
You might say: "When interacting with sales clerk, client exhibited anxiety and required 2 verbal cues to relax."

Rather than saying: "Child was asked a series of yes/no questions"
You might say: "Child responded to yes/no questions correctly 20% of the time."

Deemphasize the Treatment Media

In order to improve a client's performance skills, OTAs often use various media, such as equipment or activities that will help the client reach functional goals. However, when recording observations of these treatment sessions, the OTA should deemphasize the media used and focus instead on the performance skills being addressed. For example, an inexperienced OTA might write the following:

"Client worked on placing pegs into a pegboard."

This sentence may accurately describe what a casual observer would see, but as a trained professional the OTA needs to look beyond the media used and see what the client was really accomplishing. The treatment media used here are pegs and a pegboard, but what is the performance skill? Placing pegs into a pegboard is not a practical skill a client needs in order to be able to care for himself; however, the performance skill practiced during this activity may well be crucial to achieving independence. Suppose the OTA had written:

"Client worked on tripod pinch using pegs and a pegboard."

Notice that in this example the OTA did not simply add the performance skill to the statement *"Client worked on placing pegs into a pegboard to increase tripod pinch"* but actually turned the sentence around so that the tripod pinch received the emphasis and the treatment media was mentioned only for clarification. Suppose that the OTA had written:

"Client worked on tripod pinch in order to be able to grasp objects needed for ADL tasks."

In this case, mention of the media becomes optional. The OTA might also have written:

"Client worked on tripod pinch using pegs and a pegboard in order to be able to grasp objects needed for ADL tasks."

Which of the three preceding examples do you think best describes the skilled occupational therapy instruction that is occurring in this treatment session? This may seem like a minor distinction, but it is very important in demonstrating the need for skilled occupational therapy and the emphasis on functional outcomes in therapy.

One of the most common errors that inexperienced OTAs make is focusing on the media used, rather than on the performance skill that is being improved by use of the media. Consider this OTA's observation:

Client was seen in rehab center for standing balance activities. Client stood to walker with min Ⓐ for balloon toss. Client used Ⓡ UE to hit balloon and was able to reach to Ⓡ and Ⓛ sides approximately 7 out of 10 tries. Activity was continued for 3 minutes. Client requested rest break and sat for 30 seconds. Client then stood with mod Ⓐ to walker and hit balloon with Ⓛ UE for 3 minutes. Client was able to hit balloon approximately 6 out of 10 times and spontaneously switched to Ⓡ hand x2 when balloon was to her far right. Client sat for another break and to switch activities. Client stood CGA to toss beanbags with Ⓡ hand for 4 minutes. Client scored 240 points with Ⓡ hand by throwing beanbags at target. Once all beanbags were thrown, client sat for a 30-second break. Client stood with CGA for balance to toss beanbags with Ⓛ hand for 30 seconds. Client scored 150 points with Ⓛ hand by throwing bean- bags at scoring target. Once all beanbags were thrown, client sat and session was ended.

When this note is rewritten to focus on the performance skills instead, notice the significant difference in professionalism in the way the note reads:

Client seen in clinic for dynamic and static standing balance activities needed for ADL and IADL tasks. Client stood to walker with mod Ⓐ for dynamic standing balance necessary for Ⓘ showering using a balloon toss activity. Client held walker with Ⓛ hand and used Ⓡ UE to reach both Ⓡ and Ⓛ sides approximately 7/10 attempts. Client sustained activity for 3 minutes continuously and then took a 30- second rest break. Client stood to walker again with mod Ⓐ for 3 minutes of continuous activity involv- ing weight shifting and balance required in balloon tossing. Client demonstrated ability to reach to Ⓡ and Ⓛ sides for moving object approximately 6/10 times. Client demonstrated ability to spontaneously shift weight 2 times to reach object. Client took 30-second rest break before next activity. Client worked on dynamic standing balance using beanbag toss activity with target. Client stood to walker for 4 min- utes of dynamic balance activity with CGA, then sat for 30-second rest. Client stood again with CGA for 3 1/2 minutes of continuous dynamic balance activity.

Worksheet 7-1
Deemphasizing the Treatment Media

Rewrite the following statements to concisely emphasize the skilled occupational therapy that is actually occurring in the intervention session:

1. *Client played a game of catch using bilateral UEs to facilitate grasp and release patterns.*

2. *Resident put dirt into pot to halfway point, added seedling, and filled remainder of pot with dirt which was transferred by cup. Resident completed 3 more pots while standing 8 minutes before requiring a 5-minute rest. Resident then resumed standing position for approximately 5 minutes to water completed pots.*

3. *Client painted some sungazers in crafts group in order to be able to see that she could do something successfully.*

Make Certain That It Is Clear That You Were Not Just a Passive Observer in the Session

This will be a critical factor in reimbursement. OTAs do not just get paid to watch a client do something. To demonstrate that the skill of an occupational therapy practitioner is needed, you must be actively involved in intervention, such as assessing or modifying the activity; otherwise it will be considered unskilled.

Rather than saying: "Client compensated for shoulder flexion by leaning forward with whole body during prehension activities."
You might say: "Client required skilled instruction to avoid compensation at the shoulder during prehension activities."

Rather than saying: "Client performed home exercise program."
You might say: "Home exercise program was observed for accurate movement patterns and updated to accommodate for progress."

Although You Will Assess the Information You Observed and Make a Professional Judgment About It, Avoid Judging the Client

Rather than saying: "Client was compliant" or "Client was cooperative."
You might say: "Client demonstrated ability to follow 3-step directions and sequence WFL."

When working with a client who exhibits difficult personality traits or behavior, or whose opinions you do not agree with, it is easy to judge the client and to reflect your judgments in your observation. However, you must be careful to maintain your professional attitude and avoid personal or emotional judgments. Below is an example of a note written by an OTA who was experiencing a difficult client situation. The client "went off on" the OTA. The client refused to get out of bed, lied about having already performed grooming tasks, threw her toothpaste on the floor, refused to brush her teeth or comb her hair, and cursed at the OTA. In spite of all this, the OTA wrote an observation that was nonjudgmental of the client:

Client initially declined grooming tasks but after max encouragement demonstrated ① supine → sit on EOB c̄ good dynamic sitting balance to perform grooming. Client ① brushed hair and teeth with use of bedside table and set up. Client ① retrieved toothpaste tube from floor using a reacher. Client expressed frustration regarding her illness by saying several profane words.

Be Specific About Assist Levels

When giving assist levels, be sure to note what specific aspect of the activity the client needed assistance or verbal cues to perform. For example:

*Veteran doffed night garment with min Ⓐ to **untie strings on back**.*

*Pt. able to sequence steps to prepare cup of tea but required verbal cue to **turn off stove**.*

*Child needed HOH assist **for accuracy** when cutting with scissors.*

*Client required verbal cues **to sit down** in order to doff hosiery.*

*Consumer able to follow bus schedule with min verbal cues to **identify correct time.***

*Patient stand → w/c using a standard walker with min physical Ⓐ and min verbal cues **to bring walker completely back to w/c.***

*Infant able to roll supine to prone with min tactile cues **to initiate movement.***

*Client required mod Ⓐ **to follow total hip precautions** while using long-handled sponge for washing lower legs and feet.*

In trying to be concise, sometimes inexperienced OTAs make the mistake of writing an "**O**" that contains only a list of actions with assist levels. Although this is a common error, it is **incorrect**. Simply writing a list of activities or assist levels does not demonstrate that skilled OT is being provided. Consider this OTA's observation:

Client was seen for 1 hour in the shower room to ↑ activity tolerance and improve balance during showering, and was shown a smaller shower which simulated her home shower, in order to prepare for discharge in one week.
Client OX4.
Client min Ⓐ with verbal cues to sit in w/c to doff hosiery and to dry off LE.
Client spontaneously rinsed soap off hands before gripping grab bar while showering.
Client used walker going to and coming from shower room.
Client tolerated standing Ⓘ during entire shower.
Client instructed in home showering.

Now look at the same observation rewritten in a more useful format below:

Client was seen for 1 hour in the shower room to ↑ activity tolerance and improve balance during showering and was also shown a smaller shower which simulated her home shower, in order to prepare her for Ⓘ and safe showering after discharge in 1 week.

Mobility: Pt. walked to/from shower room Ⓘ and safely with the aid of a standard walker to provide stability in shower room while dressing/undressing.

Cognition: Client oriented X 4.

BADL: Client min Ⓐ with verbal cues to sit down in order to doff hosiery and to dry LEs safely. During shower, client spontaneously rinsed soap off hands prior to gripping grab bar s̄ verbal cues. Client tolerated standing Ⓘ ~ 5 minutes during shower s̄ SOB. Skilled instruction provided in safe technique to use in her single shower stall and recommendations given re: grab bar placement.

Worksheet 7-2
Being Specific About Assist Levels

When noting assist levels in your observation, it is not enough to note only the level of assistance required. You must also note the **specific part** of the task that required assistance. For example:

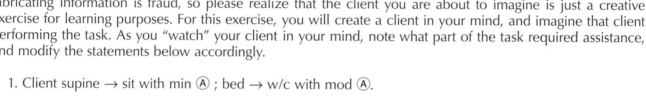

*Resident donned pants with min Ⓐ to **pull up over hips**.*

*Student able to operate power w/c c̄ **min verbal cues and use of wrist splint to operate joystick**.*

*Client propelled w/c from room to OT clinic but required verbal cues **to avoid running into other clients**.*

Rewrite the statements below to indicate a **part** of the task that required assistance. Since you have not seen the client, you cannot really know what part required assistance. In the usual world of professional behavior, fabricating information is fraud, so please realize that the client you are about to imagine is just a creative exercise for learning purposes. For this exercise, you will create a client in your mind, and imagine that client performing the task. As you "watch" your client in your mind, note what part of the task required assistance, and modify the statements below accordingly.

1. Client supine → sit with min Ⓐ ; bed → w/c with mod Ⓐ.

2. Client required SBA in transferring w/c ↔ toilet.

3. Client retrieved garments from low drawers with min Ⓐ.

4. Brushing hair required max Ⓐ.

5. Client completed dressing, toileting, and hygiene with min Ⓐ.

Use Standardized Terminology and Grade Your Treatment Activities

It is important to qualify and quantify the level of assistance required and the complexity of the activity demands. If you write, *"Resident required assistance to don upper and lower extremity garments,"* that doesn't give the full picture. Did the resident require supervision, minimal assistance, moderate assistance, or maximal assistance? Was the supervision close or distant, constant or intermittent? Did the resident require cues? If so, how many cues and what kind: physical, verbal or visual? Did the resident use compensatory methods or adaptive devices? Were there safety issues, problems with performance skills or client factors?

Also consider the activity demands in order to document the grading and adapting of your treatment activities. For example, the activity requirements are easier for donning slip-on shoes rather than shoes that require tying. Perhaps, instead, the patient uses shoes with hook and loop closure or elastic laces. Pants with elastic waistbands are easier to don than pants that require fastening with a button and zipper. Did the client don a front button shirt or a pullover shirt? A front closure, back closure, or pullover bra? Try to be as specific as possible with the activity demands. For the previous example, it would be better to say:

> *Resident required min Ⓐ and 3 verbal cues to place elastic waist pants over affected lower extremity with use of reacher while sitting on EOB. Resident then donned slip on shoes with supervision and verbal cue for task initiation. CGA required for balance to stand and pull up pants. Resident donned front closure bra with min Ⓐ to fasten. Pullover sweater donned with verbal cue required to identify front/back of sweater.*

Another example would be a home management task such as preparing lunch. Instead of saying, *"Client Ⓢ in preparing lunch,"* it would be better to describe the type or complexity of lunch that the client prepared:

> *Meal preparation skills assessed. Client required supervision to prepare a simple microwave lunch (TV dinner). Client able to read and follow package directions, open package, and use microwave. Required 2 verbal cues to handle hot food safely.*

Table 7-2 presents some suggestions for grading and describing kitchen tasks for documentation, along with some examples. You may come up with other categories. For each meal preparation task, consider the activity demands such as number of steps involved, level of complexity, performance skills, and client factors required. Note if the task involves safety issues, reading directions, opening packages, measuring, use of tools or appliances, clean-up, and time management.

Table 7-2.

Graded Levels of Meal Preparation

- Obtain a snack (get yogurt or fruit from refrigerator, cheese and crackers)
- Simple cold meal preparation (cereal and milk, sandwich)
- Cold meal preparation involving safety/tool use (salad, tuna fish)
- Microwave snack or meal (popcorn, frozen dinner, soup)
- Toaster or toaster oven (toast, waffles, frozen pizza)
- Simple stovetop task (tea, soup)
- Min complex stovetop (grilled cheese, pudding, scrambled eggs)
- Mod complex stovetop (tacos, macaroni and cheese)
- Complex meal (follow a recipe, 2-, 3-, 4-course meal)

You can apply these principles to other activities such as home management tasks. Consider the activity demands of light household chores (folding towels, wiping a table, dusting) vs. heavy household chores (mopping a floor, washing windows, and changing sheets). Also, if the client uses an ambulation device or wheelchair for functional tasks, the specific type of device should be noted. While not an all-inclusive list, some types of ambulation devices and wheelchairs are listed below:

- Crutches
- Single point cane
- Quad cane
- Hemi-walker
- Standard walker
- Rolling walker
- Platform walker
- Standard wheelchair
- Power wheelchair
- Bariatric wheelchair
- Sip and puff wheelchair

Remember that as an OTA you are not issuing ambulation devices or simply instructing the client in ambulation or gait training. That is most likely considered physical therapy and would be duplication of services or possibly beyond your scope of practice. Rather, in occupational therapy, your focus is on **safe functional mobility for specific occupational tasks**. You might say:

Resident required min Ⓐ to get clothes out of closet while standing with rolling walker.

Student required min verbal cues and CGA to obtain items on bottom of locker with use of crutches and a reacher.

Child was able to use platform walker safely to navigate in bathroom, transfer on/off toilet, and manage clothing for toilet hygiene.

Client required CGA with use of quad cane to load dishwasher.

Helpful Hint

Good documentation is based on accurate observation, which is based on knowing what to look for. For an experienced professional, this becomes second nature. For an OTA student, it is helpful to review the lists in this manual and to check your observations against what your supervising therapist observed during the treatment session to be sure you are noticing the items that matter most.

You have now completed the "**O**" part of your note. As you can see, it is extremely important for the OTA to focus on function, communicate skilled services, and accurately describe and record activity demands and client performance. The next chapter will address the third section of the SOAP note—the assessment.

Chapter 8

Writing the "A"—Assessment

The third part of the note is the **ASSESSMENT**. This section consists of the occupational therapy practitioner's skilled appraisal of the client's progress, functional limitations, pertinent issues and expected gains from rehabilitation. In the assessment section of the note, you will use your professional judgment to discern the meaning of the data you have presented in the "**S**" and the "**O**" sections. You will also relate how this data will impact on the client's ability to benefit from occupational therapy and engage in meaningful occupations.

For example, during the intervention session, you may have observed that the client does not attend to the left side. Perhaps you observed that he only ate food on the right side of his meal tray and he couldn't find the toothpaste tube or brush on the bathroom counter. You will note both the problem (left neglect) and the areas of occupation in which it is a problem (basic ADL tasks). In your assessment, to address the impact of this deficit, you might write:

> *Left neglect interferes with ability to perform BADL.*

In the assessment section of the note, the OTA will remark on the 3 P's: **problems, progress,** and rehab **potential**. The OTA might also identify and explain inconsistencies, discuss emotional components, consider contexts or new issues, or present some reason that something was not implemented or achieved as planned.

Assessing the Data

To assess the data, go **sentence by sentence** through the data presented in the "**S**" and the "**O**." For each component, consider the implications for the client's engagement in meaningful occupational activities and role performance. Note what problems, progress, or rehabilitation potential you surmise. Consider these possibilities:

Problems May Include the Following

Safety Risks
- *Safety concerns noted when child attempted to stand without locking brakes on w/c.*
- *Poor problem solving when using the stove raises safety concerns.*
- *Client's poor short-term memory limits ability to adhere to THR precautions.*
- *Client's limited coping strategies for dealing with stress raise concerns for continuing the use of self-destructive behaviors.*

Factors Not WFL That Can Be Influenced by Occupational Therapy Intervention

- Left side weakness interferes with standing balance in tub.
- Left side neglect necessitates verbal cues to attend to left side during BADL tasks.
- Deficits in cognitive processing create a need for constant verbal cues to perform kitchen tasks safely.
- Continued verbal threats toward other clients indicate a need for anger management techniques.
- Right hand pain and edema limit client's ability to perform heavy household chores.
- Lack of voluntary wrist and finger extension limits child's ability to engage in developmental play activities.
- Lack of spatial orientation to identify letter shapes interferes with ability to learn to read.

Inconsistencies Between Client Report and Objective Findings

- Although client reports anticipating no difficulty in returning to driving, her left-side neglect and hemianopsia would cause significant safety risks.
- Although the client expresses a willingness to perform ADL tasks, sequencing and motor planning problems create barriers to tasks.
- Although the client expresses a desire to regain skills for return to work, he has not followed through with his home exercise program and has missed several occupational therapy appointments.
- Client verbalizes a desire to progress to the next level of responsibility, but shows ↓ behavioral control when reward incentives are unavailable.
- Although student expresses a desire to improve handwriting, student has not followed through with use of thumb stabilization splint and built-up pen.

Progress Remarks May Indicate One or More of the Following

Verification That the Treatment Being Provided Is Effective

- Weighted utensils decrease intention tremors by ~ 50% when eating.
- Spouse demonstrates good carryover in ability to transfer client safely.
- Gains in prehension skills this week now enable client to button shirt Ⓘ.
- Patient has shown progress since the beginning of the week by demonstrating the ability to follow 1-step commands 80% of the time during ADL tasks.
- Client's spontaneous participation in group discussion shows good progress in developing social interaction skills.
- Infant's UE strength is increasing as demonstrated by ability to maintain prone on elbows.
- Child's progress from 70% to 90% accuracy in shape recognition indicates good recall.
- Pt. demonstrates good carryover in care and use of protective splint.

Statements That Previous Goals Have Been Met or Changed

- STG #2 (transfer to toilet with min assist) met this week.
- STG #3 upgraded to "stand at sink for 10 minutes to perform grooming tasks."
- STG #4 changed to "initiate conversation with peer during craft group."

Reasons for the Lack of Progress

- *Student has become more dependent in transfers this week 2° medication change resulting in ↑ tone in Ⓑ LEs.*
- *Patient has become more dependent in ADL tasks this week due to acute infection.*
- *Client has been unable to follow through with home program due to death of spouse.*
- *Resident has had increased difficulty feeding herself this week 2° recent wound in dominant hand.*

Potential for Success in Rehabilitation

- *Patient's intact sensation and presence of voluntary movement demonstrate good rehabilitation potential.*
- *Client's ability to recognize stressors shows good potential to change self-destructive coping strategies.*
- *Student's improvement from 50% to 60% accuracy with typing words using mouthstick indicates good potential to meet goals stated in IEP.*
- *Patient's ability to recall and demonstrate 3/3 hip precautions shows good potential to follow hip precautions after discharge.*

Writing the Assessment

As you carefully and systematically review the material in your "**S**" and "**O**", you might find it helpful to create a quick list of things to discuss in the "**A**" section of your note. For example, consider the following "**S**" and "**O**":

S: Client stated his dominant right hand "feels clumsy." He also reported difficulty with managing clothing fastenings.

O: Client seen in OT clinic for remediation of fine motor skills and hand strengthening for ADL performance. Client worked on three point and lateral pinch with use of button board and clothespins. He was issued lightly resistive therapy putty and was instructed in home exercise program. Written copy of exercises also provided and client demonstrated all exercises accurately. Client was issued a buttonhook with built-up handle. He demonstrated ability to use buttonhook to fasten and unfasten small buttons Ⓘ following instruction. Client expressed satisfaction and willingness to continue use of buttonhook and putty at home.

The following areas of progress/problems/potential can be identified:

Problems

Client is concerned regarding deficits in hand function.
Client is still unable to manage fastenings independently.

Progress

Client is able to understand and integrate therapy tasks.
Client is able to use adaptive equipment to compensate for ADL deficits.
Client is willing to follow through with home program.

Potential

By using professional judgment, the OTA would consider the client's progress shown thus far a good indicator of rehabilitation potential. The assessment of the data can then be written as follows:

A: Client's ability to accurately demonstrate exercises and use of buttonhook indicates good rehab potential. Client appears motivated and able to follow through with home program.

Justifying Continued Treatment

One very useful way of justifying continued OT treatment for your client is to end the "A" with the statement *"Client would benefit from. . ."* Then, based on your observations and assessment, complete the sentence with a justification of continued treatment that requires the skill of an occupational therapy practitioner. Not every OT or OTA ends the "A" in this fashion, but for purposes of learning, we will end the "A" with this method. This helps to make certain that justification for continued treatment is present in the note, and is a good way to set up the plan. As you become more proficient in writing notes and are confident that your note justifies continued treatment, you may choose to cover this material in the plan instead. Below are some examples:

- *Resident would benefit from environmental cues to orient him to environment.*

- *Child would benefit from assistive technology to perform classroom tasks.*

- *Client would benefit from ultrasound and TENS to ↓ hand pain to enable return to work.*

- *Parent would benefit from further instruction in positioning child for feeding.*

- *Consumer would benefit from continued instruction in problem solving and anger management techniques needed for successful personal and social relationships.*

- *Client would benefit from continued skilled OT to improve decision making skills and time management to ↓ self-destructive behaviors.*

- *Client would benefit from further instruction in total hip precautions in order to safely manage IADL tasks.*

- *Infant would benefit from activities that encourage trunk rotation to facilitate rolling over.*

- *Client would benefit from reacher, sock aid, and long-handled shoe horn to minimize low back pain when performing lower body dressing.*

- *Resident would benefit from skilled instruction in sequencing of tasks to increase safety while performing toilet hygiene and bathing tasks.*

- *Client would benefit from instruction in energy conservation and work simplification techniques to perform meal preparation and cleanup.*

Justifying Continuation of Services

When you justify the need for continuation of occupational therapy services, it is also necessary to document the reason the service must be provided by an occupational therapy practitioner rather than by another professional (e.g., PT, SLP) or nonprofessional (e.g., aide, volunteer). Consider the specialized skills and services that occupational therapy practitioners provide.

Occupational Therapists, With Contributions from the Occupational Therapy Assistant, Provide the Following Services (AOTA, 2005c)

- Evaluate clients, identify problems, establish goals, and develop intervention, transition, and discharge plans
- Assess or reassess the effectiveness of adaptive equipment, compensatory techniques and therapeutic activities in order to modify the intervention plan

Occupational Therapists and Occupational Therapy Assistants Provide the Following Services (AOTA, 2004b)

- Modify and adapt activities, functional tasks, and environmental contexts such as workstations, classrooms, and homes to enable occupational performance
- Modify activities through the provision, instruction, and use of adaptive equipment/assistive devices/technology
- Teach adaptive and compensatory techniques
- Facilitate and improve developmental skills
- Fabricate/modify/instruct in use of splints, orthotics, prosthetics, and adaptive devices
- Provide individualized, specialized, and skilled instruction to the client/family/caregiver
- Promote psychosocial health
- Determine the safety and effectiveness of performance skills, task procedures, and equipment
- Intervene to address safety hazards, unsafe, and at-risk behaviors
- Improve performance skills and client factors through remediation approaches
- Administer physical agent modalities as a means to facilitate occupational performance (AOTA, 2003b; AOTA, 2004b)

Specific Types of Skilled Occupational Therapy Instruction to the Client, Family, or Caregiver Might Include (AOTA, 2004b)

- Instruction in individualized therapeutic exercise programs
- Instruction in the development or remediation of specific life skills for occupational roles and contexts
- Instruction in coping mechanisms, behavior management, assertiveness training, strategies for stress or anger management
- Instruction in specific leisure, social, and interpersonal skills
- Education regarding community services and support systems
- Instruction in energy conservation and work simplification
- Instruction in joint protection
- Driver rehabilitation and education
- Instruction in body mechanics and ergonomics
- Instruction in prevocational and vocational task skills
- Instruction in positioning of the limbs, trunk and head to facilitate ADL, and address client factors such as normalizing tone, reducing edema, and facilitating safe swallowing

Skilled Occupational Therapy Is **Not** Evident When the OT or OTA Provides the Following Services

- Provides unnecessary or unreasonable services for a client who cannot tolerate interventions, has poor potential to meet rehabilitation goals, or who is expected to spontaneously recover a transient loss of function such as after a general surgery (CMS, 2005e)
- Carries out diversionary activities or groups not appropriate or relevant to the intervention plan (CMS, 2005e)
- Duplicates services with another discipline or provides services that unskilled personnel are able to do (CMS, 2005e)
- Continues routine interventions or maintenance programs such as self care activities, passive range of motion, or monitoring of exercise programs after the adapted procedures are in place, outcomes are reached, or no further significant progress or changes are expected or needed (CMS, 2005e)
- Provides services that are not part of an occupational therapy intervention plan (CMS, 2005e)
- Has a patient watch a video or read a handout such as for ergonomics or body mechanics without providing skilled instruction or practice of the skills (CMS, 2005e)
- Administers routine physical agent modalities without relating them to performance of occupational tasks (AOTA, 2003b)

Wording is critical to documenting the necessity for continuing skilled occupational therapy. The occupational therapy practitioner **provides skilled instruction** to clients rather than **assisting** them. For example, an occupational therapy practitioner may provide instruction in methods of energy conservation and work simplification rather than help the client perform a strenuous task. OTs and OTAs collaborate to **design** and provide **instruction** in home programs, which will then be carried out by aides, caregivers, and family members. Why should a third party payer reimburse you to watch a client carry out the home exercise program that he performs daily on his own? However, if you are **assessing** his ability to do all the components of it correctly, or **modifying** it to compensate for recent progress, then your professional skill as an OTA is clearly required.

Analyze your clinical reasoning and then document the principles and strategies used during an intervention session in justifying the continuation of skilled occupational therapy. Billing insurance companies for unjustified services or falsifying documentation is unethical and may be considered fraud or abuse with severe legal implications. Also, if you state that the client will benefit from further specific occupational therapy interventions, you must be prepared to follow through with this. Remember that the justification for continued occupational therapy treatment must support the frequency and duration of the plan. If the last sentence of your "A" reads, *Client would benefit from information on energy conservation techniques*, do not expect the payer to approve more than one more treatment session unless that you indicate that functional training and practice is required for implementation.

If this is your last session, complete the sentence with the OT's discharge plan (that you as the OTA may also have contributed to). For example:

Client would benefit from continued PROM provided by caregiver.

Client has been instructed in home safety modifications and she would benefit from the installation of bathroom grab bars.

Client would benefit from Meals on Wheels to eliminate need for grocery shopping.

Student would benefit from continued participation in peer support group.

Client would benefit from continued use of home paraffin and TENS unit PRN for pain.

Ending the Assessment

Now we can finish the assessment section of the note we began earlier:

S: Client stated his dominant right hand "feels clumsy." He also reported difficulty with managing clothing fastenings.

O: Client seen in OT clinic for remediation of fine motor skills and hand strengthening for ADL performance. Client worked on three point and lateral pinch with use of button board and clothespins. He was issued lightly resistive therapy putty and was instructed in home exercise program. Written copy of exercises also provided and client demonstrated all exercises accurately. Client was issued a buttonhook with built-up handle. He demonstrated ability to use buttonhook to fasten and unfasten small buttons Ⓘ following instruction. Client expressed satisfaction and willingness to continue use of buttonhook and putty at home.

describes activity

*A: Client's ability to accurately <u>demonstrate exercises</u> and use of buttonhook indicates good rehab potential. Client appears motivated and able to follow through with home program. **Client would benefit from** further instruction in adapted equipment, compensatory techniques, and remediation of fine motor skills in order to regain Ⓘ in all ADL.*

Here are some more examples of what the completed assessment section of your note might look like for other practice settings:

A: Client is beginning to regain some of the independent living skills she had prior to her recent psychotic episode. Fear, isolation, and ↓ activity tolerance slow her progress and are the focus of current treatment. Client would benefit from continued skilled instruction in self-care skills as well as ↑ socialization and ↑ physical activity.

A: Child's poor attention span and inability to tolerate auditory stimuli limit her ability to control her classroom behavior. She would benefit from more activities to ↑ tolerance of auditory stimuli and strategies to manage self-control.

New Information

The assessment section is **not** the place to introduce new information. Do not put anything in your "A" that has not already been discussed in the "S" or "O." If you find yourself wanting to make a statement in the "A" that is not supported by the data in your "S" or "O," ask yourself what you might have observed to support the assessment statement. Then decide whether you need to add it to your "S" or "O."

<u>Helpful Hint</u>

The assessment section demonstrates your clinical reasoning as an OTA and is the "heart" of your note. If you could write only six lines, the assessment section of your note would contain the six lines you would choose.

Worksheet 8-1
Justifying Continued Treatment

Which of the following requires the skill of an OTA?

_____   Administering paraffin irrelevant to occupational performance.

_____   Instructing the client in leisure skills for stress management.

_____   Having a client watch a video on assertiveness training without further instruction or without role-playing the techniques.

_____   Analyzing and modifying functional tasks/activities through the provision of adaptive equipment, or techniques.

_____   Determining that the modified task is safe and effective.

_____   Carrying out a maintenance program.

_____   Upgrading a strengthening program.

_____   Teaching the client to use the breathing techniques he has learned while performing his ADL activities.

_____   Interpreting initial evaluation results and establishing the intervention plan.

_____   Providing individualized instruction to the client, family, or caregiver.

_____   Giving the patient a replacement piece of hook and loop fastener.

_____   Providing specialized instruction to eliminate limitations in a functional activity.

_____   Developing a home program and instructing caregivers.

_____   Teaching compensatory skills.

_____   Gait training.

_____   Making skilled recommendations to a parent for a child's positioning and feeding.

_____   Educating clients to eliminate safety hazards.

_____   Presenting information handouts (such as energy conservation) without having the client perform the activity.

_____   Routine exercise and strengthening programs.

_____   Adding instruction in lower body dressing techniques to a current ADL program.

_____   Teaching adaptive techniques such as one-handed shoe tying.

Now you can try to integrate the information in this chapter. Review the following occupational therapy note:

S: Client says she has difficulty moving ® UE, although she does not know why it will not move. She reports "It really doesn't hurt. It's just tight."

O: Client seen in rehab gym for UE activities to ↑ AROM in ® shoulder, activity tolerance, UE strength, and dynamic standing balance, in order to ↑ independence in ADL activities.

BADL: Client seen in room for instruction in safety techniques and adaptive equipment use in toileting. Client required use of bilateral grab bars in bathroom to sit → stand safely. Client first attempted to stand while pulling on walker and one grab bar. Client instructed on safety issues and the use of bilateral grab bars.

Performance skills: Client sit → stand CGA for balance. Client worked on activity tolerance, dynamic standing balance and ↑ AROM in right shoulder by moving canned goods from counter to cupboard for 5 minutes before needing to sit and rest 2 minutes. She then participated in activities to ↑ dynamic standing balance by pouring liquid from a pitcher while standing CGA for balance. After a 1-minute rest, client continued activities to ↑ dynamic standing balance and safety in ADL activities by pushing wheeled walker while picking up objects from the floor with a reacher.

Client factors: AROM in right shoulder abduction <90°. PROM right shoulder abduction WNL.

Think about how you would you assess this information. Review the suggestions given earlier in the chapter, and then organize your thoughts by identifying the problems, progress, and rehabilitation potential you see in this client's treatment session today. What problems and safety risks can you identify? Are there performance skills and client factors not WFL that occupational therapy might impact? Do you see any evidence of progress or rehab potential? What would this client benefit from? Identify problems, progress, and rehab potential using Mini-Worksheet 8-2. Then compare your ideas with the suggested assessment that follows.

Mini-Worksheet 8-2: Organizing Your Thoughts for Assessment

Problems

Progress

Potential

In preparing an assessment of the data in this note, two main **problem** areas can be determined: the safety of transferring to and from the toilet, and the client factors that were not WFL. The OTA should be particularly concerned about the safety issues, and those should be addressed first. Also, the OTA should note the rehabilitation **potential** that would help a reviewer to decide whether the client's progress is sufficient to warrant the expense of treatment.

A: *Safety concerns (impulsivity, ↓ dynamic standing balance) noted when client attempts to transfer sit → stand during toileting. Client verbalized an understanding of safety instructions and has potential to progress to independence.*

Next, the OTA should note the clinical reasoning behind devoting time to addressing client factors, considering the client's rehabilitation potential.

A: *Safety concerns (impulsivity, ↓ dynamic standing balance) noted when client attempts to transfer sit → stand during toileting. Client verbalized an understanding of safety instructions and has potential to progress to independence.* **Client's ↓ AROM in right shoulder, ↓ activity tolerance, and ↓ dynamic standing balance all interfere with ability to complete ADL tasks safely and independently.**

The OTA can then complete the assessment by justifying continued treatment.

A: *Safety concerns (impulsivity, ↓ dynamic standing balance) noted when client attempts to transfer sit → stand during toileting. Client verbalized an understanding of safety instructions and has potential to progress to independence. Client's ↓ AROM in right shoulder, ↓ activity tolerance, and ↓ dynamic standing balance all interfere with ability to complete ADL tasks safely and independently.* **Client would benefit from Ⓡ UE AROM and strengthening exercises along with continued skilled instruction in safety issues and energy conservation techniques.**

In this case, the OTA can address client factors in two different ways, both by working on ↑ AROM, strength, and activity tolerance, and by teaching some energy conservation strategies.

Third party payers often deny ongoing treatment of range of motion and strength. Occupational therapy practitioners must consider the expected functional gains vs. the costs of continuing treatment. Clinical decisions must be made to determine if a home exercise program could accomplish the same results or if skilled services remain appropriate and necessary. In Chapter 9, you will see how an OTA can cost-effectively provide the proper interventions to benefit this client.

Assessing Factors Not Within Functional Limits

Every note does not necessarily reflect **progress** and/or rehabilitation **potential**. However, most notes do indicate **problem** areas. This is because the problems are what limit occupational performance and necessitate client treatment. The most common problem area that the OTA assesses is the impact of an underlying limiting factor such as a performance skill or client factor that is deficient. When OTA students and novice clinicians are first learning to write SOAP notes, they may find it difficult to distinguish observations from assessments. This can also sometimes cause notes to be redundant. There is a helpful formula to address a problem area that is not WFL. This will ensure that you are actually writing an assessment rather than an observation. State the limiting factor at the beginning of the sentence, and then describe or relate how that factor impacts a client's functional ability in a particular area of occupation.

Underlying Limiting Factor	Functional Impact	Ability to Engage in Occupation

For example:

- ↓ **oral motor control** interferes with child's ability to manage solid foods.

- **Edema and ↓ ROM in dominant hand** limit client's ability to perform child care tasks.

- **Inability to self-regulate alcoholic intake** results in difficulty maintaining employment.

- ® **shoulder pain** interferes with client's ability to perform sliding board transfers and propel w/c.

- **Deficits in short-term memory, attention span, and problem solving** make meal preparation tasks unsafe.

The subject of the sentence in each of the above examples reflects the performance skill or client factor that is not WFL. What follows next is the negative influence it has on a specific area of occupation. This method is useful when you are first learning, but do realize there can be other ways to write assessment statements.

Worksheet 8-3
Assessing Factors Not WFL

Use the following formula to rewrite the assessment statements and make them more effective.

Underlying Limiting Factor	Functional Impact	Ability to Engage in Occupation

For example, this statement is an observation:

Client's activity tolerance for standing at the stove was < 4 minutes 2° inability to tolerate prosthesis.

It tells you the client behavior and measurable factors the OTA can observe while providing intervention. To make it into an assessment statement, you would need to change the emphasis by turning your sentence around and by adding the impact the client's standing tolerance has on her independence in cooking. Using the formula above you might write:

Client's activity tolerance for standing with prosthesis for < 4 min limits performance of kitchen tasks.

Rewrite the following statements using the formula given above:

1. Child wrote poorly due to immature pencil grasp and difficulty $\bar{c}$ spatial orientation of letters.

2. Client demonstrated difficulty with balancing her checkbook due to memory and sequencing deficits.

3. Client experiencing manic episode and was unable to attend and follow directions for cooking activity.

4. Client problem solved poorly while performing lower body dressing as evidenced by multiple attempts to button pants and don socks.

Worksheet 8-4
Social Skills Worksheet

Your client is a middle-aged woman presently diagnosed with bipolar disorder. In a prior admission, however, she was diagnosed with schizophrenia. One of her goals is to talk to the mental health center staff about her problems rather than acting out her feelings. Today she was seen in an occupational therapy social skills group with five other clients who also need help with relationship issues.

S: Client reports that she understands the purpose of social skills group. She expressed a desire to attend all the groups, saying that they are "fun."

O: Client seen on the unit for a group session on friendship. Client appeared unkempt, with hair not combed and shirt rumpled. Client engaged in conversation with the other clients and the facilitator. Client interrupted others on five occasions. Client spontaneously verbalized her experiences with past friendships and her ideas of useful ways to make new friendships, but had to be redirected to the topic twice during discussion.

What problems are evident in the above "S" and "O"?

What areas of occupation are affected by these problems?

What evidence of progress and/or potential do you see?

Write your assessment below:

A:

Chapter 9

Writing the "P"—Plan

The final section of a SOAP note is the **PLAN**. In this section, you determine and set forth the specific treatment that will be used to achieve the occupational therapy goals. You will record what follow-up is required, such as what you plan to do in the client's next occupational therapy session or what needs to be addressed in the near future. The plan might also be a recommendation that you want the client, family, or caregiver to follow through with such as: attend a support group, install grab bars, wear a splint for work tasks, or try out a home exercise program. The plan in your SOAP note must follow the OT's intervention plan (containing long- and short-term goals, frequency and estimated duration of treatment) that was established from the initial evaluation. It should also relate to the information that you just presented in the "O" and the "A," and to your skilled assessment of what the patient would benefit from.

The plan will inform the reader of your priorities regarding intervention strategies. In a contact note or a progress note, you will address any part of the plan that has not been covered in the last sentence of your assessment, "Client would benefit from…." You will address how often the client will be treated, how long intervention will continue, and your priorities for what you will work on next or follow up with. In this book, you will learn to end the "P" with a goal. This is not the only correct way to write a plan, but it is the one we will be using. Some facilities do not include goals in this section but, instead, may only update and include new goals in reevaluation notes. The choice of what kind of goal to use depends on the individual facility. In a practice setting where notes are written monthly, your goal would be what you hope to accomplish in the next month. In an acute care setting, it might be your goal for tomorrow. In a school setting, it might be a goal to accomplish by the end of the school year. Goals are always written in measurable, objective, behavioral terms, and include a function and a time line. It is not necessary to repeatedly state goals that are already written in the initial evaluation.

Your goals in the "P" section should reflect specific task components or steps towards meeting the overall goals in the initial intervention plan. Use the format below to develop goals for your plan. If your facility does not require goals in this section, then just eliminate the last sentence in the examples below. Developing skills for goal writing will be further addressed in Chapter 11.

Client will _____ _____ _____
　　　　　　(action verb—what will client do)　　　(skill)　　　(how or under what conditions)

_____　　_____ .
(for what function or occupational gain, if not already indicated)　　(time frame—by when)

Examples of a "**P**" might include:

Consumer to be seen for 2 more weeks for 60 min, twice weekly sessions for skilled instruction in performing IADL. By anticipated discharge on 9/13/06, consumer will be able to ① manage all laundry tasks at laundromat.

Consumer will continue prevocational program 5 days/wk. in order to ↑ task behaviors for work. Consumer will ① punch time card with one verbal cue by the end of next tx. session.

Student will continue OT 3 x wk for 30 min sessions in order to ↑ perceptual and fine motor skills for better classroom performance. Student will be able to use loop scissors to cut a straight dotted line ① within ¼ inch 3/4 opportunities by the end of the school year.

Continue one hour daily sessions for two weeks to improve motor planning skills for dressing. By the end of next session, veteran will demonstrate the ability to identify front and back of shirt with one verbal cue.

Client will continue to be seen in values clarification groups 3x wk. for 2 weeks to address low self-esteem and self-destructive behaviors. Pt will demonstrate awareness of self-help strategies by verbalizing 3 behaviors to ↓ at-risk behaviors within two group sessions.

Helpful Hint

If for some reason you are not able to see your client as scheduled, the "plan" section of your note should allow another occupational therapy practitioner to continue treatment uninterrupted.

Determining the Plan

Now let us determine the plan for the note that we assessed in the last chapter. As you recall from Chapter 8, this client has deficits in safety and standing balance.

S: Client says she has difficulty moving right UE, although she does not know why it will not move. She reports "It really doesn't hurt. It's just tight."

O: Client seen in rehab gym for UE activities to ↑ AROM in ® shoulder, activity tolerance, UE strength, and dynamic standing balance, in order to ↑ independence in ADL activities.

ADL: Client seen in room for instruction in safety techniques and adaptive equipment use in toileting. Client required use of bilateral grab bars in bathroom to sit → stand safely. Client first attempted to stand while pulling on walker and one grab bar. Client was instructed on safety issues and the use of bilateral grab bars.

Performance skills: Client sit → stand CGA for balance. Client worked on activity tolerance, dynamic standing balance and ↑ AROM in right shoulder by moving canned goods from counter to cupboard for 5 minutes before needing to sit and rest 2 minutes. She then participated in activities to ↑ dynamic standing balance by pouring liquid from a pitcher while standing CGA for balance. After a 1-minute rest, client continued activities to dynamic standing balance and safety in ADL activities by pushing wheeled walker while picking up objects from the floor with a reacher.

Client factors: AROM in right shoulder abduction <90°. PROM right shoulder abduction WNL.

A: Safety concerns (impulsivity ↓ dynamic standing balance) noted when client attempts to transfer sit → stand during toileting. Client verbalized an understanding of safety instructions and has potential to progress to independence. Client's ↓ AROM in right shoulder, ↓ activity tolerance, and ↓ dynamic standing balance all interfere with ability to complete ADL tasks safely and independently. Client would benefit from Ⓡ UE AROM and strengthening exercises along with continued skilled instruction in safety issues and energy conservation techniques.

Write your plan for this client below. Begin with a statement about how often (once or twice daily, 2x wk, etc.) and for how long (for 3 days, for 2 weeks, for 1 month, etc.) she will be treated. Look at the items indicated above that she would benefit from, and set your priorities. End with a correctly written goal to be accomplished in the next treatment session.

Mini-Worksheet 9-1: Determining the Plan

P:

Completing the Plan

In assessing the data, the OTA has set up the plan for this note. The OTA has already justified the main intention and indicated the client's rehabilitation potential. Now the OTA needs to be specific about how often the client will be treated and for what length of time. This will reflect the frequency and duration of treatment that the OT initially established in the intervention plan. Some facilities do not restate the frequency and duration in every subsequent treatment note but we will write the plan this way.

P: Continue to treat client 5x wk. for 1 week...

The OTA could have specified the length of the treatment sessions, e.g., **for 1 hr. sessions**, but chose not to do that in this particular note. Next the OTA specifies how the treatment time will be used:

P: Continue to treat client 5x wk. for 1 week **for skilled instruction in safe transfers and toileting**.

Since discharge is anticipated in 1 week, the OTA must prioritize treatment time in order to implement the OT's intervention plan. As the OT has delegated treatment of this client to the OTA, the OTA might choose in this case to work on balance and energy conservation as a part of functional mobility and ADL activities. Since the OTA has already written that the client would benefit from additional AROM and strengthening exercises, there now needs be a specific note of how these needs will be addressed.

P: Continue to treat client 5x wk. for 1 week for skilled instruction in safe transfers and toileting. **Home program for AROM and strengthening exercises for Ⓡ shoulder will be taught**.

This OTA has also indicated clinical reasoning in planning for discharge in advance of the discharge date. When providing feedback to the OT and recording later notes, the OTA will indicate the client's progress in learning the home program. Simply handing the client a set of printed exercises is not considered a billable service. The client's progress in learning the home program will also confirm the OTA's assessment that the client's rehabilitation potential was on target. The OTA will end this plan with a measurable, action-oriented, time-limited goal. Notice that the OTA has specified the conditions under which this action will be carried out.

P: Continue to treat client 5x wk. for 1 week to work on safe transfers and toileting. Home program for AROM and strengthening exercises for ® shoulder will be taught. **Client will be able to Ⓘ demonstrate HEP and will also spontaneously use bilateral grab bars during toilet transfers by the end of next session.**

This note is now complete.

Numbering the Short-Term Goals

Some occupational therapy practitioners number each short-term goal. For example:

STG #1: Consumer will Ⓘ select and insert correct amount of money in coin-operated washing machine by 8/25/06.

STG #2: Consumer will Ⓘ select proper cycles on washing machine by 8/25/06.

In subsequent notes, the clinician can refer to those numbered goals, providing a clear indication of the progress achieved. For example:

A: STG #2: met. STG #1: Consumer requires min verbal cues 50% of the time to select proper wash cycles for white and dark clothes.

P: Consumer will continue skilled instruction in IADL until anticipated discharge in 4 weeks. At the time of discharge, consumer will be able to manage all laundry tasks Ⓘ at laundromat.

Worksheet 9-2
Completing the Social Skills Plan

As you recall from Chapter 8, your client is a middle-aged woman diagnosed with bipolar disorder. In a prior admission, however, she was diagnosed with schizophrenia. One of her goals is to talk to the mental health center staff about her problems rather than acting out her feelings. Today she was seen in an occupational therapy social skills group with five other clients who also need help with relationship issues. The assessment's last sentence indicates some areas of intervention that might benefit this client. Now try to fill in the specifics of the plan.

S: Client reports that she understands the purpose of social skills group. She expressed a desire to attend all the groups, saying that they are "fun."

O: Client seen on the unit for a group session on friendship. Client appeared unkempt, with hair not combed and shirt rumpled. Client engaged in conversation with the other clients and the facilitator. Client interrupted others on five occasions. Client spontaneously verbalized her experiences with past friendships and her ideas of useful ways to make new friendships, but had to be redirected to the topic twice during discussion.

A: Client's unkempt appearance, interrupting behaviors, and need for redirection to topic of conversation interfere with her ability to engage in social participation with peers. Her expressed interest in groups, her willingness to engage in conversation and share her ideas show good potential to develop relationships and to express herself verbally in place of acting out. Client would benefit from attending groups stressing conversational skills and attention to social cues, and from assistance with ADL activities stressing hygiene and appearance.

P:

Worksheet 9-3
Completing the Plan: Additional Practice

Now try to finish the plan section for the following note. Think about what you would need to follow up with. Also consider what other specific interventions or adaptive equipment might help this client.

S: Client stated his dominant right hand "feels clumsy." He also reported difficulty with managing clothing fastenings.

O: Client seen in OT clinic for remediation of fine motor skills and hand strengthening for ADL performance. Client worked on three point and lateral pinch with use of button board and clothespins. He was issued lightly resistive therapy putty and was instructed in home exercise program. Written copy of exercises also provided and client demonstrated all exercises accurately. Client was issued a buttonhook with built-up handle. He demonstrated ability to use buttonhook to fasten and unfasten small buttons ① following instruction. Client expressed satisfaction and willingness to continue use of buttonhook and putty at home.

A: Client's ability to accurately demonstrate exercises and use of buttonhook indicates good rehab potential. Client appears motivated and able to follow through with home program. Client would benefit from further instruction in adaptive equipment, compensatory techniques, and remediation of fine motor skills in order to regain ① in all ADL.

P:

Chapter 10

Special Situations and SOAP Analysis

Special Situations

There are special situations that require documentation even if the client wasn't seen face to face or didn't receive a complete occupational therapy session. Sometimes sessions get cancelled for various reasons or unusual circumstances may occur. Besides recording these situations, you should document any necessary communication or follow-up regarding these events. This will ensure coordination of care and also help protect you should any legal issues arise later on. You must also record the date, time, and sign the note. Here are some examples:

Refusals and Cancellations

Sometimes a client might refuse or cancel occupational therapy services either completely or only for one particular session. Always document the refusal or cancellation and indicate the reason why whenever possible.

Client refused OT today because he felt "dizzy and nauseous." Nursing was notified.

Student went on class trip and, therefore, was unable to receive OT today.

Patient called to cancel OT appointment because his car broke down. Appointment was rescheduled for tomorrow.

Patient cancelled his OT initial evaluation and stated he does not want any therapy. Patient was educated regarding the reason for referral and benefits of OT but pt. still refused services. MD was notified.

Attempted to see client today but client was unavailable due to medical test procedures (X-ray and MRI). Will attempt to see client again tomorrow.

Father called to cancel child's appointment because child has a stomach virus.

Client called crying and stated she was cancelling OT today because of her agoraphobia. She reported having a severe anxiety attack this morning and was fearful of leaving her home. Pt. also reported her medication made her "feel worse." Attempted to reassure pt. and advised her to contact her psychiatrist to discuss her anxiety and medication issues. Encouraged client to attend next OT session scheduled in 2 days.

No Shows

Sometimes a client has an OT appointment and simply does not show up.

Pt. did not show up for appointment. Call made to pt.'s home; he stated he forgot appointment. OT rescheduled for tomorrow.

No show. Attempted to call pt. but no one answered the phone.

Child did not show up for appointment. When parent was contacted by phone, she stated she couldn't get the time off from work today. Appointment was confirmed for next OT session in 2 days.

Client did not show up for appointment. Call made to pt.'s home. Pt. stated he could not "get motivated" to get out of bed and get dressed due to "very depressed mood." Client did not express suicidal ideation and stated he was adhering to his medication regime. Client also stated that he realizes OT is important for his recovery and will ask his sister to bring him to tomorrow's OT session.

Resident did not show up for scheduled OT session. Called nurse's station and RN stated resident wasn't feeling well this morning and was sleeping. Will attempt to see resident again this afternoon.

Treatment Interruptions

Sometimes you are about to start an OT session or are in the middle of an intervention and the treatment gets interrupted for various reasons. Any intervention provided should be documented along with the reason for the therapy interruption.

Client was transferred from bed to w/c with min assist. Client then stated she did not feel well and vomited. Changed client's soiled garments and notified nursing staff.

Child seen in dining room for instruction in feeding skills. Five minutes into session, the physician came to take child for medical evaluation. Will attempt to see child again tomorrow for instruction in feeding skills.

Upon arrival to OT clinic, resident stated she needed to have a bowel movement. Resident was transported back to her room and nursing staff was notified.

Client arrived at OT visibly upset. She stated, "I can't go on. I really feel like killing myself." Attempted to calm pt. and contacted social worker who requested COTA bring pt. to her office immediately. Pt. was then transported to social worker's office to address her emotional status.

Medical Hold

Sometimes the patient's medical condition warrants that therapy be put on hold and this may be indicated in the physician's orders, by the nursing staff, by the therapist's discretion, or facility policy.

MD orders state pt. on hold for therapy today 2° possible blood clots in Ⓛ LE.

Nursing requested that OT be deferred today due to pt.'s side effects from chemotherapy.

Upon arrival to OT clinic, pt. stated she fell yesterday on her affected ® UE. Right hand is now moderately edematous and bruised and pt. reports severe pain. Clinician immediately called MD who requested OT be put on hold until MD evaluates pt. to determine ® UE status. Pt. advised to follow up with physician ASAP.

OT deferred today due to child having surgery for insertion of feeding tube.

Pt. called to report he was hospitalized for two nights 2° pneumonia. OT deferred until physician's orders received to resume OT.

Client on hold as per MD orders 2° to psychotic episode.

Incidents

Sometimes accidents or incidents happen no matter how careful you are. Each facility should have specific policies and procedures on how to document and handle incidents regarding staff, clients, visitors, or volunteers. Protocols are usually in place to deal with safety, security and medical issues, standard precautions, proper notification of superiors, administrative follow through and liability issues. Often, there are separate incident report forms to fill out besides the information that is recorded in the health record. Only report the actual facts. **Learn the exact policies and procedures in your facility so you are prepared to handle any incidents promptly and properly**.

Upon COTA's arrival at pt.'s room, pt. was found lying on floor crying. Nursing staff and physician were immediately notified.

Upon arrival at OT cooking group client suddenly picked up a pan and hit himself on the head with it, sustaining a bruise. Client was immediately removed from cooking group and taken to nurse's station for evaluation of self-inflicted injury.

Client sustained a small cut to left small finger while cutting vegetables in cooking group. Wound cleansed and bandage applied. Nursing notified.

Child became angry when told he must stay seated in his chair. He then yelled several profane words and bit clinician's hand. Child was then sent to principal's office to address inappropriate behavior.

As an OTA, you must always be prepared to react quickly and appropriately to unexpected circumstances. Obtain the most knowledge you can in regards to facility policies, emergency procedures, first aid, infection control, pertinent laws, and current occupational therapy practice, so you will be prepared. When special situations and unusual circumstances do arise, you must always use professional judgment, maintain your professional demeanor, and keep the OT informed. Document in a timely manner, avoid judgments, report the facts carefully and accurately, and do what is in the client's best interest. Before we begin looking at other types of occupational therapy notes, complete the following worksheet to review the mechanics of documentation that you learned in Chapter 2. Remember that certain basic elements or guidelines must be present in all documentation formats. The rest of this chapter will present additional tips for analyzing and recording your observations during treatment.

Worksheet 10-1
Mechanics of Documentation

Look at the following contact note and see how many elements you can find that are incorrect or missing. Realize that this note reflects a "special situation" and, therefore, does not need to include the complete S, O, A, and P format.

XYZ School District
Albany, NY

John Doe

3/22/06   Upon arrival to OT room, student reported he had a headache, felt nauseous, and said he was "burning up." OT session defered and student escorted to ~~teach~~ nurse's office.

C. Caring, COTA

1.

2.

3.

4.

5.

6.

7.

8.

9.

10.

Improving Observation Skills

It is important to hone your observation skills and organize your thoughts in order to document intervention sessions appropriately and accurately. As indicated in previous chapters, you will make numerous observations during a treatment session while professionally assessing the client's responses, behavior, task performance, and issues related to his condition. You will then have to document these professional observations so someone reading your note will get a clear mental picture of the client's situation and what transpired during the intervention session. If possible, jot down observations and information during the therapy session or as soon as possible. This will help you to remember pertinent facts when you later organize the information into a SOAP note. As you gain clinical proficiency and develop your own repertoire of professional terminology, it will become easier over time.

Here are some additional questions and tips to consider during client interventions. Use these suggestions to improve your observation skills and help organize information for your SOAP notes.

WHO Is Involved in the Treatment Session?

- Are family members, caregivers, or other staff present or involved in the treatment session?
- Is your client interacting with other clients?
- Is this a group activity?

WHEN Did the Treatment Take Place?

- Did you treat the client during a specific mealtime, during morning self-care, after dinner, during a classroom activity, group session, etc.?
- What did the client do just before your treatment session and will this impact his performance in OT? For example, perhaps the client just underwent a strenuous medical treatment or just had physical therapy, which is the reason why the client is now tired, doesn't feel well, or performs poorly.

WHERE Did the Treatment Session Take Place?

- Did you work with the client bedside, in the emergency room, OT clinic, ICU, classroom, outdoors, in a group session, home visit, or in the community?
- Did you perform ADL in the kitchen, bedroom, bathroom, dining room, or other area?
- Did you transfer or ambulate the client from one place to another and, if so, did the client require any equipment such as grab bars, a trapeze, Hoyer lift, or ambulation device?
- Did the client remain in bed, in a wheelchair, geri-chair, or regular chair the entire session and did you use any positioning devices such as a laptray, arm rest, supports, or cushions?
- Did the client stand or sit at a desk, kitchen table, counter, bathroom sink, mat, computer workstation, or other surface?

WHAT Happened During the Treatment Session?

- What did the client, caregiver, family, or staff members say or ask?
- What functional activities did the client do and what skilled services did you provide to address the client's goals?
- What techniques, equipment, or modifications were used or provided, such as adaptive equipment, weights, therapy putty, worksheets, games, splints, or physical agent modalities?

- Were any measurements taken or specific skills assessed in this treatment session?
- What instruction did you provide to the client, family, caregiver, or staff?
- What abilities, limitations, problems, safety concerns, or progress were evident during the therapy tasks?
- What will you need to follow-up with?

WHY Is the Particular Treatment Intervention Important?

- Why is this particular treatment relevant to the client's intervention plan and goals?
- Why is the treatment activity a skilled service that required the expertise of an occupational therapy practitioner?
- Why did the patient have a particular outcome during this session?

HOW Did the Client Perform or Participate in the Task?

- How does the treatment plan need to be modified based on this treatment session?
- How were problems or issues handled?
- How is the client progressing?
- How did the client, family, caregiver, or staff respond, react, or perform during this intervention?

The following worksheets will enable you to incorporate the above suggestions with guidelines from the prior chapters. This will allow you to begin making observations and use your clinical reasoning skills for writing your own original SOAP notes. You are now one step closer to becoming an OTA.

Worksheet 10-2
Improving Observation Skills

Try an activity with a classmate to improve your observation and documentation skills. Realize that this is simply a creative role-playing exercise.

Pretend your partner has had a stroke and cannot use the dominant upper extremity. Pick an ADL to work on (e.g., putting on a shoe or jacket, making a sandwich, etc.) and teach your partner compensatory techniques, just as you would a client. Now, using the suggestions in this chapter as a guide, list the following:

WHO

WHAT

WHERE

WHEN

WHY

HOW

Using this information, now write a SOAP note regarding your partner's "treatment session" on a separate page.

Worksheet 10-3
Improving Observation Skills—More Practice

Now try another activity with a classmate to improve your observation and documentation skills. Realize that this is simply a creative role-playing exercise.

Pretend your classmate has arthritis or COPD and has decreased upper extremity AROM and difficulty performing ADL. Pick one ADL to work on (e.g., cooking, grooming, managing fastenings) and teach joint protection, energy conservation or compensatory techniques. Also, teach your partner some exercises to improve AROM. Then, use the suggestions in this chapter to list the following:

WHO

WHAT

WHERE

WHEN

WHY

HOW

Using this information, now write a SOAP note regarding your partner's "treatment session" on a separate page.

Chapter 11

Goals and Interventions

Occupational therapy goals must be written in functional, measurable, observable, action-oriented terms. They must be realistic for the client, appropriate for the practice setting, and able to be achieved in a reasonable amount of time. Goals are initially formulated in the OT's intervention plan and must reflect the functional outcomes that the client hopes to gain from occupational therapy. Although improving underlying client factors or biomechanical components may be essential to achieving the functional outcome, these are much less important to a third party payer than what the client can actually do. The OTA will implement day-to-day treatment activities to achieve the functional outcomes outlined in the intervention plan. What transpires during the intervention session is recorded in a SOAP note. As you learned in Chapter 9, the "P" part of the SOAP note often ends with a goal. You will be aligning your treatment to the established intervention plan and will write goals to reflect the steps along the way that your client needs to achieve desired outcomes.

Goals

Goals in an intervention plan are also called **long-term goals** (LTG) or outcomes. These are usually discharge goals—what the client hopes to accomplish by the time of discharge. For each problem the OT has identified, there will be at least one long-term goal, and often more than one.

Objectives

Objectives are also called **short-term goals** (STG). These are the incremental goals that are met while progressing toward the discharge goals. For example, if the long-term goal is:

In order to perform job without injury, client will be able to move 35# objects needed for work from table to counter without ↑ in pain by 9/18/06.

then a short-term goal might be:

In order to perform job tasks, client will be able to lift 10# objects needed for work without increase in pain by 9/5/06.

Figure 11-1. Steps to the Ultimate LTG.

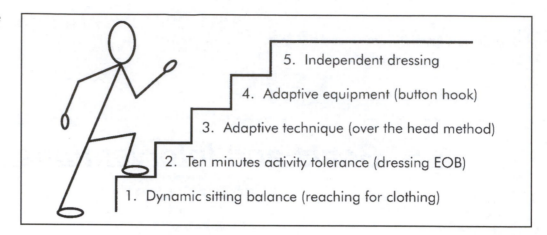

5. Independent dressing

4. Adaptive equipment (button hook)

3. Adaptive technique (over the head method)

2. Ten minutes activity tolerance (dressing EOB)

1. Dynamic sitting balance (reaching for clothing)

There may be several short-term goals (objectives) for each long-term goal. For example, suppose you are treating Mr. H., a 49-year-old mailman who sustained a Ⓡ CVA a few days ago and has Ⓛ side hemiplegia. The OT's evaluation states that he has verbal abilities and intact mental functions. The intervention plan has identified a goal of independent upper body dressing by 7/21/06. This will require skilled instruction and the correct adaptive equipment.

A series of objectives must be established:

1. In order to begin dressing activities, client will be able to maintain dynamic sitting balance at edge of bed for >5 minutes while reaching for clothing at arm's length by the end of the 3rd treatment session.

2. By the 6th treatment session, client will be able to tolerate > 10 minutes of dressing while sitting at edge of bed.

3. After skilled instruction, client will be able to don shirt sitting EOB using the over the head method by 7/15/06.

4. After skilled instruction, client will be able to button shirt Ⓘ c̄ use of a buttonhook by 7/18/06.

5. While sitting on edge of bed, client will be independent in upper body dressing by 7/21/06.

As you can see, each of these short-term goals is measurable, observable, and action-oriented. The first four short-term goals are steps to reach the ultimate long-term goal (Figure 11-1).

An intervention plan is always a work in progress and you and the OT will collaborate to provide the most appropriate care. Unexpected events and conditions can impact the progress your client will be able to make toward his or her goals. The OT will modify the intervention plan as needed (based upon your feedback), as it is not useful to continue with a plan that is not working. In order to write appropriate goals and objectives in a way that can be measured, the elements to be included are very specific. The FEAST format (Table 11-1) is useful as you are learning to write goals, although the order may need to be changed slightly in order for your sentence to make sense. As long as all the required elements are present, you can begin with any of the FEAST elements—the expectation, the conditions, the timeline, the functional outcome.

Now let us look at each category a little more closely.

F (Function)

This is the specific area of occupation to which this goal pertains, if it is not already imbedded in the goal, for example, "in order to return to work as a carpenter," "in order to be able to be bathed by his caretakers," or "in order to be able to write his name at school." Here is an example:

In order to begin writing his name at school, the student will demonstrate ability to hold a crayon using tripod pinch by 9/19/06.

Table 11-1.
Goal Writing: The FEAST Method
F – Function   → For what occupational gain? E – Expectation   → The client will... A – Action   → Do what? S – Specific Condition → Under what conditions? T – Timeline   → By when?

The function may go after the action if you prefer. For example:

The student will be able to hold a crayon using tripod pinch in order to learn to write his name at school by 9/19/06.

Often the function is the same as the action.

The client will perform a three-step cooking process at wheelchair level by 9/16/06.

In this case, the function (cooking) is inherent in the goal so there is no need to restate it. Function is the ability to engage in occupation, and is the heart and core of occupational therapy practice. It should be the **first** thing you think of when writing goals, and should be the essential focus of the goal statement.

E (Expectation)

In writing treatment goals, the client is the key player. The occupational therapy practitioner sets the expectation:

The client will . . .

Note: These are the client's goals. The goal statement is **not** the place to tell what the therapist will do. That goes later, under intervention strategies. In some instances, the goal might indicate what the parent or caregiver will achieve after your skilled instruction:

*After skilled instruction, **parent will** demonstrate proper technique to position child for feeding by end of 2nd treatment session.*

***Client's spouse will** demonstrate ability to safely transfer client from bed ↔ commode following skilled instruction within 1 week.*

A (Action)

An action verb is inserted here such as perform, demonstrate, initiate, identify, cook, don, transfer, comb, unfasten, or complete, followed by the skill to be performed. For example:

*The client will **perform a three-step cooking process.***

In this case, the function is contained in the action statement, and therefore does not need to be added.

S (Specific Condition)

This is the level of assistance expected and/or the conditions under which the client is expected to be able to perform the desired action. For example: "...after set up"; ". . .by using a reacher"; ". . .at wheelchair level"; "while standing at sink"; ". . .after skilled instruction."

*The client will perform a three-step cooking process **at wheelchair level**...*

The conditions make your goal more specific. Usually it is helpful to put the condition **after** the skill rather than before it, but sometimes you may want to start with the condition. For example:

***After skilled instruction** the client will be able to perform a three-step cooking process...*

Below are some examples of goals in which the conditions have been highlighted for emphasis. One of the most common mistakes in goal writing is omission of the conditions under which the activity is expected to be performed.

Examples

*In order to dress herself with minimum assistance, client will ① button at least three buttons on her shirt **using a buttonhook** by 10/1/06.*

*In order to be able to begin skilled instruction in dressing by 9/30/06, client will maintain static sitting balance ① on **edge of bed** for 3 minutes.*

*In order to demonstrate increased self-esteem, client will verbalize three positive attributes **with min verbal prompting** within 1 week.*

T (Timeline)

This is the time frame within which the goal is expected to be accomplished. For example "...by discharge on 10/16/06," "...by the end of the next treatment session," or "...within 2 weeks".

*The client will perform a three-step cooking process at wheelchair level **by 10/16/06**.*

Documentation must demonstrate a clear need for skilled occupational therapy, as you learned in Chapters 1 and 8. Once a client reaches the level of minimal assistance, the changes become more subtle, and may lead to denial of payment unless you specify the necessity of skilled occupational therapy. For example, dressing with minimal assist does not necessarily indicate a need for skilled occupational therapy. However, "minimal assistance with verbal instruction for over-the-head compensatory method of donning shirt" justifies skilled occupational therapy.

Educational Goals

Occupational therapy practitioners working in the public schools use a slightly different terminology. In education, goals for one school year are called "objectives." Educational goals are not measured by time, e.g., *by 5/7/06* or *"within 3 weeks."* Since the IEP is rewritten annually, the time frame for educational goals is assumed to be annual. Children sometimes exhibit a new behavior inconsistently before it is really established. Therefore, measurement used for children is more likely to reflect whether or not the behavior is established.

For example:

Kevin will hold pencil in a tripod grasp in 3/3 opportunities.

Chrystal will demonstrate improved tolerance to tactile media as evidenced by self-initiation during art activities in 5/5 teacher reports.

Student will demonstrate ability to open combination lock on locker while getting to next class on time 4/5 opportunities.

   You may find that some school settings use percentages in goals such as *Child will demonstrate ability to bring food to mouth with spoon without spilling 75% of the time by the end of school year.* However, it is more clear to say *Child will demonstrate ability to bring food to mouth with spoon without spilling 15/20 opportunities by the end of school year.* This way anyone can observe the exact behavior, number of repetitions, and determine if the criteria are met. Goals for children in the public schools must be set in terms of a behavior that is needed in the classroom or school context. While you may be working on sensory integration as a treatment intervention such as maintaining prone extension posture over a therapy ball, it must be written in language that is educationally based, relating to performance in the classroom setting.

Student will maintain upright sitting posture during writing time without verbal reminders in 3/3 observations.

DO NOT use participation in treatment as a goal. For example:

Client will do 20 reps of shoulder ladder with 1# wt. in order to ↑ endurance to become more ⓘ in ADL.

In a goal such as this, specify the amount of ↑ endurance you hope or expect to see. For example:

Client will be able to participate in assembly line task > 10 minutes without rest breaks.

Rather than saying: Client will use therapy putty to ↑ hand strength by 5 lbs.
It is better to say: Client will ↑ hand strength by 5 lbs. in order to be able to open jars.

Rather than saying: Client will play a board game with other clients.
It is better to say: Client will demonstrate improved self-confidence by ⓘ initiating a leisure activity with peers.

Examples of Appropriate Goal Statements for Different Situations

Basic Activities of Daily Living

Dressing
- Child will be able to manage zipper on coat with use of zipper pull within 1 month.
- In order to tie shoelaces ⓘ, patient will demonstrate Ⓡ thumb MP flexion of no less than 50° within 2 weeks.

Hygiene

- Patient will complete grooming and hygiene activities with a reported pain level of < 3/10 within 3 tx. sessions.
- Student will be able to perform feminine hygiene Ⓘ by end of school year.
- Client will demonstrate 10 min activity tolerance for standing at sink to brush teeth, comb hair, and shave within 4 tx. sessions.

Eating/Feeding

- Resident will feed self a meal with correct use of adaptive equipment (nonslip placemat, lipped plate, rocker knife, and built-up angled utensils) after set-up with no more than one 5 minute rest break within 30 days.
- Consumer will choose at least two food items other than pizza that he is willing to include in his diet within 1 week.

Functional Mobility

- In order to return to living at home, patient will be able to propel w/c up ramp and through all doors with min Ⓐ within 2 weeks.
- In order to grocery shop Ⓘ, consumer will explain the bus schedule including which stops she commonly uses within 2 weeks.

Instrumental Activities of Daily Living

- In order to return to living unassisted, patient will demonstrate an ability to prepare a min complex stovetop meal Ⓘ after the 4th treatment session.
- In order to manage laundry Ⓘ, client will correctly sort white and dark clothes by next treatment session.

Education

- In order to complete writing activities, Steve will be able to maintain upright posture at desk for >5 minutes without verbal cues within 6 weeks.
- Child will be able to open combination lock on locker Ⓘ 4/5 trials by the end of school year.

Work

- Consumer will Ⓘ request a job application from a restaurant within 1 week.
- In order to return to carpentry work, patient will demonstrate Ⓡ UE grip strength > 70# within 4 weeks.

Play

- In order to engage in developmental play activities, child will sit unsupported for 3 minutes within 2 months.
- Leroy will use Ⓛ UE as a functional assist 5/5 opportunities during spontaneous play within 2 months.

Leisure

- Client will identify at least three leisure activities that are not associated with drinking by 10/8/06.
- Within 1 month, client will demonstrate sufficient coordination to manipulate toothpaste caps, clothing fastenings, and knitting needles without dropping.

Social Participation

- Consumer will choose and participate in at least one social activity per week 3/3 weeks within 1 month.
- With mod verbal cues, consumer will ask roommate to smoke outside the building.

Worksheet 11-1

Evaluating Goal Statements

Determine which of the following goals have all the necessary FEAST components to be useful in occupational therapy documentation. For each goal that is incomplete or inaccurate in some way, indicate what it lacks.

1. *By the time of discharge in 1 week, client will be able to dress himself with min Ⓐ for balance using a sock aid and reacher while sitting in a wheelchair.*

   ___ This goal has all the necessary components to be useful.

   ___ This goal lacks _____

2. *Client will tolerate 15 minutes of treatment daily.*

   ___ This goal has all the necessary components to be useful.

   ___ This goal lacks _____

3. *Client will demonstrate increased coping skills in order to live at home with her granddaughter within 2 weeks.*

   ___ This goal has all the necessary components to be useful.

   ___ This goal lacks _____

4. *Resident will demonstrate 15 minutes of activity tolerance without rest breaks using Ⓑ UE in order to complete self-care tasks before breakfast each morning.*

   ___ This goal has all the necessary components to be useful.

   ___ This goal lacks _____

5. *In order to be able to toilet self Ⓘ after discharge, client will demonstrate ability to perform a sliding board transfer w/c → mat within the next week.*

   ___ This goal has all the necessary components to be useful.

   ___ This goal lacks _____

6. *OTA will teach lower body dressing using a reacher, dressing stick and sock aid within 2 tx. sessions.*

   ___ This goal has all the necessary components to be useful.

   ___ This goal lacks _____

7. *In order to return to living independently, patient will demonstrate ability to balance his checkbook.*

   ___ This goal has all the necessary components to be useful.

   ___ This goal lacks _____

Worksheet 11-2

Writing Functional, Measurable Goals

Review the scenarios below and write measurable, functional, and time limited goals that are realistic for these situations. Goals are established with the client (under the supervision of the OT), so assume for this practice sheet that you have already collaborated regarding the client's goals.

1. Your client, Maria, has difficulty with IADL tasks because she is unable to attend to task for more than a few minutes. Since she enjoys cooking and plans to resume cooking after discharge, you have been working with her in the kitchen. You would like to see her able to attend to task for 10 minutes by the time she is discharged next week. Write a goal to increase Maria's attention span.

F (if not included in action) _____
(For what functional gain)
E _____
(Expectation—the client will)
A _____
(Action)
S _____
(Specific Conditions)
T _____
(Time line—by when?)

2. Now write a goal for Maria to be able to follow directions so that she can read the back of a boxed meal, and eventually a recipe, when she is cooking.

F (if not included in action) _____

E _____

A _____

S _____

T _____

3. Bill is having trouble performing dressing tasks after his stroke. In occupational therapy, you have been teaching him an over-the-head method for putting on his shirt, and have given him a buttonhook to use. Write a dressing goal for Bill.

F (if not included in action) _____

E _____

A _____

S _____

T _____

4. Susan has significant weakness and desires to be able to be able to care for her 4-month-old child and also go back to work as a receptionist. Write a goal to increase her activity tolerance. Anticipated discharge is in 2 weeks.

F (if not included in action) _____

E _____

A _____

S _____

T _____

5. Alberto wants to live independently in the community, but lacks basic money management skills. Write a goal for Alberto to improve his money management skills.

F (if not included in action) _____

E _____

A _____

S _____

T _____

6. Katelyn has become increasingly more depressed over the past several weeks, and was admitted after a suicide attempt. You estimate that you will have her in groups for 1 week. You would like to see her mood change in that week. Write a goal that will indicate an improved mood.

F (if not included in action) _____

E _____

A _____

S _____

T _____

Worksheet 11-3

Writing Functional, Measurable Goals: Developmental Disabilities

Jake is an 18-year-old male with developmental disabilities. He has just moved into a group home with five other clients. Jake exhibits mild to moderate cognitive impairment but can perform personal ADL with supervision and occasional assistance. Muscle tone is minimally hypotonic but there are no other physical limitations. He has a fair frustration tolerance and occasionally exhibits some aggressive behavior. The plan is to improve Jake's social skills and allow him to be more independent in the home and community.

Using the information in the above scenario, write a short-term goal for each of the areas of occupation listed below. Make sure your goals are appropriate and realistic for this particular practice setting, keeping in mind the client's abilities and expected functional gains.

Instrumental ADL—meal preparation _____

_____

Instrumental ADL—household chore _____

_____

Instrumental ADL—shopping _____

_____

Instrumental ADL—money management/functional math skill _____

_____

Communication/Interaction skills _____

_____

Prevocational skills _____

_____

Temporal organization/Time management _____

_____

Chapter 12

Evaluation and Intervention Planning

Referral Process

As we discussed in Chapter 1, occupational therapy practitioners write different kinds of notes for different stages of the intervention process. The process begins when a client is referred to occupational therapy. Each agency has its own policies and procedures to facilitate the referral process depending on the practice setting, licensure laws, and other ethical and legal requirements. Occupational therapy practice acts may differ from state to state regarding scope of practice (such as use of physical agent modalities) (Slater & Willmarth, 2005) and whether a prescription is required for evaluation and/or treatment. The practice acts also delineate which healthcare professionals can legally write a prescription for occupational therapy (such as a physician, nurse practitioner, or physician's assistant). Let us consider some examples of the referral process.

For an inpatient setting such as a hospital or long-term care facility, an order for occupational therapy is established in the medical record by the physician (or other appropriate professional). Depending on the facility, this entry might be initially be handwritten, or entered by computer, telephone, or other means. This occupational therapy prescription could be initiated when the client is first admitted or might be established later as the need for occupational therapy arises. The occupational therapy department is then notified of the order by procedures established by the facility such as a computer entry or a call from the unit secretary. The client is then seen by the OT as soon as possible according to established guidelines. In an outpatient setting, when a new client calls (or stops by) to schedule an appointment, the occupational therapy department will consider the urgency of the appointment (such as if the patient needs to be seen that same day) and schedule it according to the client's needs and OT's schedule. The client's diagnosis, insurance, and contact information might also be verified during that initial phone contact. The request for special services or occupational therapy in a school setting might be initiated by a parent, teacher, or other staff. The request is considered by the child study team and the child is evaluated as appropriate by the necessary disciplines. An Individualized Education Program (IEP) is then established to determine what specific services will be provided.

Regardless of the practice setting, the OT is responsible for responding to the new referral (AOTA, 2005c). We will now look at each step of the occupational therapy evaluation process.

Overview

Very early in the process, an **intake note** may be written by the OT acknowledging the referral and stating a plan to evaluate. Next, the OT writes a screening or **evaluation report** that contains the client's occupational profile, current concerns and priorities, as well as the assessment results. From this comes the **intervention plan**, technically the part of the evaluation report that outlines the specific areas of occupation to be addressed, the outcomes expected, and the particular services that will be provided in occupational therapy. An OTA can contribute to this screening and evaluation process by performing delegated assessments and providing feedback and documentation to the OT (AOTA, 2005c). Facilities vary in the type, format, and frequency of **contact** or **progress notes** required. Some settings require a **contact note** (also called a **treatment note** or **visit note**) for each visit. Others may require a progress note every week, 2 weeks, every 30 days, or more frequently for new referrals or for a change in status. Contact notes and progress notes are written by the OT or OTA (under the supervision of the OT) and often use the SOAP format you have learned in this manual. The requirements for type and frequency of notes are usually a function of the practice setting, payment source, and the accrediting agency. Sometimes a **reassessment note** is required at regular intervals. When a client is transferred from one setting to another within the same service delivery system, a **transition plan** may be written. Most facilities require a **discharge** or **discontinuation report** at the end of OT treatment. This report makes recommendations, summarizes the occupational therapy services provided, and notes changes in a client's ability to engage in meaningful occupation as a result of occupational therapy intervention. Reevaluation, transition, and discharge or discontinuation reports are the responsibility of the OT. However, the OTA may contribute to these stages of treatment by performing delegated assessments and providing feedback and documentation to the OT (AOTA, 2005c).

In actual practice, you will probably find that contact, progress, and reassessment notes have some overlap. For example, in outpatient settings the contact notes often include the client's progress from session to session. Contact notes in practice settings where the client's status may change quickly, such as acute care, may seem much like progress notes. In some ways, progress notes reassess the client's status and may sound much like reassessment notes. Notes may also be named differently or combined in some service delivery systems. However, there are established basic guidelines for each kind of note.

Take another look at Chapter 2 to review the basics of documentation (such as client and facility identifying information, standards of signature, correcting errors, etc.). It would also be useful to review the description of skilled and unskilled services in Chapters 1 and 8. These criteria are applicable to all types of occupational therapy notes. Please realize that some settings use an addressograph card to stamp the client's identifying information on each page of documentation rather than having to write out this information by hand.

In *Guidelines for Documentation of Occupational Therapy* (AOTA, 2003a), criteria for notes in three process areas are described: evaluation, intervention, and outcome. Evaluation and screening reports, along with reassessment reports, are considered **evaluations**. The **intervention process** consists of the intervention plan, contact notes (also called treatment notes or visit notes), progress reports, and transition plans. Discontinuation or discharge notes record professional activity in the area of **outcomes**. Occupational therapy practitioners must meet the often difficult challenge of providing complete, comprehensive, quality care and professional documentation within the time constraints often faced due to managed care. We will now look at documentation for evaluation and treatment planning.

Initial Evaluation Reports

The Evaluation Process

From the moment the referral is received, intervention planning begins in the mind of the OT. The client's name, age, and reason for referral will stimulate a good OT to begin reviewing in his mind the areas of occupation he is likely to assess, the areas of deficits he might expect to find, and the possible interventions he might want to use. Each client is different of course, and there will be many variations, as well as some surprises as the assessment begins. The mental preparation for *"Andrew Smith, age 68, Ⓛ CVA, evaluate and treat"* takes a therapist on a mental journey along one road of thought, whereas *"Carrie Steed, age 4, ADHD"* takes the therapist mentally down a different pathway. From day one, a good practitioner also begins discharge planning based on the client's occupational profile, prior functional level, and probable discharge placement.

One of the first steps is a review of the medical chart. This allows the therapist to better understand the client's condition, determine the direction of the interview, and decide what assessments to administer. Information obtained from the medical chart might include:

- Primary and secondary diagnoses/reason for admission/hospitalization
- Medical orders: in addition to actual orders for therapy, these might include pertinent issues such as weightbearing status, type of diet (e.g., pureed, NPO, low salt), orthopedic precautions, MET level, oxygen level, permission to get out of bed, etc.
- Medications
- Procedures or surgery performed
- Past medical history
- Medical test results such as X-rays, lab tests, MRI, neurological, developmental, or psychological tests
- Home or social situation and expected discharge plan
- Information from other disciplines such as physical or speech therapy evaluation results and goals

Data is also obtained from the client, family/caregiver, and other pertinent sources. Sometimes it might be necessary to contact the physician directly to clarify orders or discuss the client's condition or precautions. The OT determines what information is needed for the client's occupational profile. This includes focusing on the client's occupational history, determining what that client needs and wants from occupational therapy, as well as what factors impact engagement in occupation. The OT selects and administers any standardized tests or survey instruments that will help determine more exactly what underlying factors support or hinder participation in occupations. The therapist might delegate some aspects of the chart review, interview, specific assessments, or other functions to the OTA.

If the client is verbal and oriented, an interview is top on the agenda. If the client is unable to provide information, the family or other caregiver may be able to provide the necessary information instead. The occupational therapy practitioner must ask questions to determine the client's occupational profile and find out what roles are important to this client. What areas of life present the most problems? What does the client hope to gain from treatment? What results are desired by the family? What was the client able to do prior to this injury, illness, or hospitalization? What supports are available to facilitate the desired outcomes? Often, much information is gleaned from simply watching the client enter into the treatment area. Does the client guard for pain? Is a supportive family member accompanying the client? What is the quality of mobility, posture, and upper extremity motion or function? Are there obvious cognitive or perceptual problems? Formal and informal assessments will be administered based on the client's condition, practice setting, and influenced by what third party payers are looking for. These might include tests relating to areas of occupation such as the Canadian Occupational Performance Measure (COPM), Functional Independence Measure (FIM™), leisure inventory, ADL observations, or other means to assess functional skills and occupational performance. Test instruments to assess performance skills or client factors might include tests such as goniometry, a manual muscle test, motor planning, task behaviors, two point discrimination, grip and pinch strength, coordination, visual perception, developmental milestones, mental status exams, and whatever else that will provide the therapist with necessary information.

Considering the initial evaluation findings, the OT will identify and prioritize the areas of occupation and underlying factors that require attention, and develop an intervention plan. Most facilities provide a form for an initial evaluation report, and evaluation results are recorded on the form, along with observations and comments. Some specific assessments are recorded on a separate form delineated for that particular test but are still included as part of the evaluation report. Facilities sometimes use the same form for reevaluation and discharge reports so that the evaluation material does not have to be rewritten. An evaluation/reevaluation/discharge report form from Capitol Region Medical Center in Jefferson City, Missouri (Figures 12-1a and 12-1b) is presented in this chapter so that you can see what might be included on a good facility form. Because this is an acute care facility, some areas of occupation (ADL) are emphasized over others (such as social participation or play). If an initial evaluation is written as a SOAP note, this is the way information would be categorized.

S: **The interview material, background information, and occupational profile**
O: **The test results and clinical observations**
A: **The OT's professional assessment of the data presented in the "S" and the "O," often written as a problem list**
P: **Frequency and duration of planned interventions and the long- and short-term goals**

CAPITAL REGION MEDICAL CENTER
OCCUPATIONAL THERAPY
☐ INITIAL EVALUATION   ☐ DISCHARGE SUMMARY

DIAGNOSIS _____ ONSET: _____

MED. HX: _____

_____ CODE STATUS: _____

RELEVANT SURG. PROC.: _____

REFERRAL DATE: _____ DATE: _____

REFERRING PHYSICIAN: _____ MEDICARE #: _____

ACTIVITIES OF DAILY LIVING   REHAB POTENTIAL: _____

DRESSING Put on & remove the following	INDEP	SBA	MIN. ASSIST	MOD. ASSIST	MAX. ASSIST	ADAPT. EQUIP.	COMMENTS/ADAPTIVE EQUIPMENT ISSUED
front opening shirt							
pull on shirt							
underwear							
bra							
pants/slacks							
socks/hose							
shoes							
manage fasteners							
braces/splints/prosthesis							
GROOMING/HYGIENE							
sponge bath							
tub/shower bath							
shave							
comb hair							
brushing teeth							
opens jars/bottles							
make-up							
EATING							
drink from cup/glass							
feeds self							
cuts meat							

UPPER EXTREMITY ROM & STRENGTH

ROM ACTIVE LEFT	PASSIVE LEFT	ACTIVE RIGHT	PASSIVE RIGHT		STRENGTH L	R
				SHOULDER: Elevation		
				Flexion		
				Abduction		
				Horizontal Abduction		
				Horizontal Adduction		
				Internal Rotation		
				External Rotation		
				ELBOW: Flexion		
				Extension		
				Supination		
				Pronation		
				WRIST: Flexion		
				Shoulder Subluxation L R		
				UE Edema L R		
				Pain L R		

PERTINENT FINDINGS

Wears glasses _____ Dentures _____ Hearing _____

MUSCLE TONE/UPPER EXTREMITIES

Hypotonic _____ Normal _____ Hypertonic _____
Comments _____

UPPER EXTREMITY SENSATION

SENSATION	Intact	Impaired	Absent
Light touch			
Sharp/Dull			
Temperature			
Proprioception			
Stereognosis			

COORDINATION/UPPER EXTREMITIES

Tremors _____ Apraxia _____ Ataxic _____

	Impaired	WNL
Gross Motor		
Fine Motor		
9 Hole Peg Test	L	R
Grip Strength	L	R
Lateral Pinch	L	R
Tripod Pinch	L	R
Hand Dominance	L	R

ORIENTED TO:

Person _____ Place _____
Time: Month ____ Day ____ Year ____
Situation _____

COMMUNICATION/COGNITION

	YES	NO
Verbal		
Understandable		
Appropriate		
Perseveration		
Follows Simple Commands		
Reads		
Writes		

PERCEPTION

	Impaired	WNL
A. R/L Neglect _____		
B. Body Schema		
C. Discrimination		
Shape		
Size		
Color		
D. Visual Perception		
Overall Endurance WFL _____		
Fair _____		
Poor _____		

SURVIVAL SKILLS	Indep.	Min. Assist	Mod. Assist	Max. Assist
Phone Book Usage				
Money Mngmt.				
Situational Problem Solving				
Homemaking				

2,605,003 (9/99) INIT. EVAL/DISCHG. SUM. (FRONT)

Figure 12-1a. Occupational therapy initial evaluation and discharge summary form (page 1). (Courtesy of Capital Region Medical Center, Jefferson City, MO.)

HOME SITUATION:_____

LIVING ARRANGEMENTS: (PT ADDRESS) _____

HOME TYPE:_____

PRIOR FUNCTIONAL INDEP.: _____

_____

_____

LEISURE INTERESTS:_____

ADAPTIVE EQUIP.:_____

COMMENTS:_____

_____

_____

_____

PATIENT / FAMILY GOALS:_____

❑ INITIAL ASSESSMENT (PROBLEMS / STRENGTHS)   ❑ DISCHARGE STATUS OF SHORT / LONG TERM GOALS

_____

_____

_____

_____

_____

PLAN:_____

SHORT-TERM GOALS - ESTIMATED TIME TO ACHIEVE: _____

_____

_____

_____

_____

_____

❑ LONG-TERM GOALS - ESTIMATED TIME TO ACHIEVE: ❑ RECOMMENDATIONS:

_____

_____

_____

_____

_____

❑ Yes   ❑ No   **Patient has participated in evaluation process and agrees with treatment plan as stated above.**

     Therapist _____ Date_____

I have reviewed and agree with the treatment plan as stated above.

     Physician Signature _____ Date_____

2,605,003 (9/99) OT INITIAL EVALUATION/DISCHARGE SUMMARY (BACK)

Figure 12-1b. Occupational therapy initial evaluation and discharge summary form (page 2). (Courtesy of Capital Region Medical Center, Jefferson City, MO.)

You will find that facilities vary in how they organize and present the information. Forms may include checklists, grids, fill in the blanks, or contain space for narrative reports. Several different formats are used in this manual to make it clear that there is no one "correct" organizational strategy.

According to the *Guidelines for Documentation of Occupational Therapy* (AOTA, 2003a), occupational analysis is fundamental and the following criteria (with examples) should be included in an evaluation:

---

a. Client information—name/agency, date of birth, gender, applicable medical/educational/developmental diagnoses, precautions, and contraindications

b. Referral information—date and source of referral, services requested, reason for referral, funding source, and anticipated length of service

c. Occupational profile—client's reason for seeking occupational therapy services, current areas of occupation that are successful and areas that are problematic, contexts that support or hinder occupations, medical/educational/work history, occupational history (e.g., patterns of living, interests, values), client's priorities, and targeted outcomes

d. Assessments used and results—types of assessments used and results (e.g., interviews, record reviews, observations, and standardized or nonstandardized assessments), description of the client factors, contextual aspects or features of the activities that facilitate or inhibit performance, and confidence in test results

e. Summary and analysis—interpretation and summary of data as it is related to occupational profile and referring concern

f. Recommendation—judgment regarding appropriateness of occupational therapy or other services

Reprinted with permission from *Guidelines for Documentation of Occupational Therapy* (AOTA, 2003a).

In an evaluation, the "**S**" may contain all or part of the occupational profile. Based on the above guidelines, some specific areas to consider might be:

- The client's living situation—type of dwelling, architectural barriers, other household members, access to family or community services

- Roles, responsibilities, and ability to care for self, children, pets, or others

- Performance patterns—typical day, limiting behaviors

- Cultural and spiritual considerations—dietary or religious issues, personal values, customs

- Educational considerations—level of education, literacy, special skills, goals

- Occupation—paid or volunteer work, is client working now, did injury occur on the job, desire to return to work, work capabilities

- Play/leisure—opportunity and barriers regarding leisure, hobbies/interests, sedentary vs active leisure tasks

- Community mobility—methods of transportation, barriers to mobility

- Community support systems

- Social—type and level of participation, clubs/organizations, successful relationships, opportunities and barriers

Here are two examples of the "**S**":

Client reports that she was admitted after a fall that resulted in a left hip fracture. Prior to admission, she lived alone in an apartment and was ① in all activities of daily living. She is 68 years old and reports that she is a retired bookkeeper, widowed 10 years ago. She expresses a strong desire to return her own apartment. She reports that her leisure activities include baking, knitting, and going to the Senior Citizen's Club twice a week (which provides transportation). Her son, who lives in the next town, provides other transportation as needed. The client's daughter lives 400 miles away but can stay with her 2 to 3 weeks after client is discharged.

The client talked about his current symptoms and the events leading up to his hospitalization. He reports losing his job with a construction company after not reporting for work for 2 weeks due to depression, having an argument with his wife, and taking an overdose. He says that he has always "worked construction" and does not know how to do anything else. He reports concern that his former employer will not give him "a decent reference." He says he really has no leisure interests except going out "drinking with the guys after work" and sometimes going hunting in the fall.

Read the following initial evaluation report and intervention plan. Use the checklist in Worksheet 12-1 to evaluate the report against the criteria described in the *Guidelines for Documentation of Occupational Therapy* (AOTA, 2003a).

XYZ Hospital

Occupational Therapy Initial Evaluation Report

Name: Agnes H.   **Medical Record #**: 12345   **Age**: 68   **Sex**: F   **Physician**: T. Grantham, M.D.
Date of onset: 5/1/06   **Date of admission**: 5/2/06
Referral Data: Client referred by Dr. Grantham for evaluation and treatment.
Occupational Profile: Client was admitted after a fall resulting in confusion and left-sided weakness. Prior to admission, she was living alone in a one-story home and was Ⓘ in all activities of daily living. Client is a retired librarian and states she values her independence and fully intends to return to her own home. Hobbies include mostly sedentary activities such as sewing, reading, and playing cards with friends. Daughter works for United Wickets, lives 2 blocks away and is willing to visit daily and assist with transportation, but cannot provide supervision.

1° Dx: Ⓡ CVA r/o OBS   **2° Dx**: diabetes
Date of evaluation: 5/3/06   **Time**: 10:00 am
S: Client stated, "I'm doing this so I can go home."
O: Client seen at bedside and in shower room for Mini-Mental State Exam, evaluation of personal ADL tasks (toileting, dressing ↔ undressing and showering) functional mobility, and underlying factors (manual muscle test, AROM)

Bathing:	Upper body: min Ⓐ to sequence task; Lower body: min Ⓐ except max Ⓐ to reach perineal area and feet
Dressing:	Seated in chair with arms, min Ⓐ to maintain dynamic balance when bending, mod Ⓐ to initiate donning bra, and max Ⓐ to reach feet. Verbal cues needed for sequencing and environmental orientation
Toileting:	Verbal cues to flush, min Ⓐ to obtain tissue and manage clothing
Transfers:	CGA with verbal cues for safety/proper arm placement sit to stand; min Ⓐ from low surfaces
Bed Mobility:	Rolls & supine ↔ sit SBA for safety
Standing Balance:	Static: CGA
Activity Tolerance:	Fair (3) (1-5 scale) <10 min tolerance to any activity with physical/mental challenges
Motor Planning/Perception:	WFL
Cognition:	Score of 17/30 on Mini-Mental State Exam. Sequencing problems during dressing tasks noted. Client could not attach bra in back and required verbal cues to attach in front
UE AROM:	WFL for all Ⓑ UE movements except: abd, int/ext. rotation of Ⓛ shoulder
UE Strength:	Grip: Ⓡ 42 lbs. Ⓛ 21 lbs. Pinch: Ⓡ palmer 14#; Ⓡ lateral 15#; Ⓛ palmer 6 #; Ⓛ lateral 8#
Manual Muscle Test:	All movements 4/5 except Ⓛ elbow ext. 3/5, thumb opposition and abduction 3+
Sensation:	Ⓛ UE: Light touch, pain, temperature intact; stereognosis 3/5; Ⓡ UE all intact

A: Client's poor problem-solving skills (trying to doff pants prior to doffing shoes/socks and inability to initiate an alternative way to don bra) and the need for verbal cues to initiate some ADL tasks limit her ability to manage her basic and instrumental ADL activities Ⓘ. Decreased AROM and strength in the Ⓛ UE along with slow response to cognitive tasks, decreased ability to sequence tasks, decreased short-term memory are safety concerns in an independent living situation. Client would benefit from environmental cues to orient her to environment, facilitation of problem solving, and sequencing activities, and activities to increase strength in the Ⓛ UE. Rehab potential is good for modified Ⓘ in ADL activities.

P: Client will be seen for 45-minute sessions 5x wk. for 2 wks. for sequencing during ADL tasks, problem-solving strategies, activities to increase activity tolerance & strength in Ⓛ UE. Put calendar in client's room to increase orientation to month, day, and season. Evaluate ability to handle emergency situations. Client will be able to dress with SBA and < 3 verbal cues after set-up within 2 weeks.

Worksheet 12-1
Initial Evaluation Report

Review the evaluation report for Agnes H. in this chapter. For each of the following criteria, determine how well the evaluation report meets the criteria established by AOTA.

Background Data

Criteria	Compliance
Are all of the following present: name, gender, birthdate? Are all applicable diagnoses listed?	
Who referred the client to OT, on what date, what services were requested?	
What is the funding source for this client?	
What length of stay is anticipated for this client?	
Why is the client seeking occupational therapy services?	
Are there any secondary problems, pre-existing conditions, contraindications, or precautions that will impact therapy?	

Occupational History and Profile

Criteria	Compliance
Is there an occupational history/profile? Is it adequate?	
Which areas of occupation are currently successful and which are problematic?	
What factors hinder the client's performance in areas of occupation? What factors support her performance in areas of occupation?	
What are the client's priorities? What does she hope to gain from OT?	
What areas of occupation will be targeted for intervention? Do these match the client's priorities?	
What are the targeted outcomes?	

Results of the Assessment

Criteria	Compliance
What types of assessments were used?	
What were the results of the assessments?	
What client factors, contextual aspects and activity demands are identified as needing attention?	
What factors (strengths, supports) facilitate her occupational performance?	
Are there other areas that need to be assessed that are not listed?	
Is OT appropriate for this client? Why or why not?	

Intervention Planning

The "**A**," or assessment, is a summary of deficits or problems that the OT determines from the initial evaluation. It is often written as a numbered list of problems (called a problem list). Problems are defined as areas of occupation that are not within functional limits that will be addressed in treatment. Problem statements should include an underlying factor (performance skill, client factor, contextual limitation, etc.) and a related area of occupation. The best problem statements give a way of measuring the extent of the problem (such as "needs max assist" or "needs verbal cues"). Also remember that those who use our services are more than an assist level, so our statements should reflect what the client is **unable to do** or **needs assistance in doing** rather than saying that the client **is** a particular assist level. Instead of a narrative format as shown in the evaluation for Agnes H., the assessment can be written as a problem list:

Problem List

1. Client needs min to max physical assist and verbal cues to dress and bathe self due to ↓ AROM, activity tolerance, and ability to sequence the task.
2. Client's lack of orientation to environment and inability to problem solve create safety concerns with ADL and home management.
3. Client needs CGA to min assist with functional mobility and transfers 2° decreased dynamic standing balance and decreased cognitive functions.
4. Fair activity tolerance limits ability to manage BADL and home management tasks.
5. Moderately decreased left hand strength limits grip and prehension for grooming and hygiene tasks.
6. Min AROM deficits in left shoulder limit client's ability to fasten bra and wash back.

The assessment is the basis upon which the OT establishes the intervention plan. The therapist collaborates with the client (along with the family or significant other when appropriate) to prioritize the problems and establish an intervention plan to achieve desired outcomes. According to *Guidelines for Documentation of Occupational Therapy* (AOTA, 2003a), the intervention plan should include appropriate long- and short-term goals, the type of approach, methods or interventions to achieve those goals, the amount, frequency, and duration of treatment, and recommendations for other services or specialized treatments. It is oriented toward the client's quality of life and ultimate success in fulfilling life roles. The intervention plan must show the need for skilled occupational therapy and be realistic; that is, it must have a good chance of success in a reasonable period of time.

Estimating Rehabilitation Potential

Rehab potential is always stated as good or excellent for the goals the OT establishes. If it is not good or excellent for the client, then a smaller, more incremental goal must be selected. There is not much point in setting and working toward goals that do not have a good chance of being accomplished. Estimating rehab potential as guarded, fair, or poor is a red flag to reviewers and they may be reluctant to set aside healthcare dollars for someone who is not likely to benefit from occupational therapy services. Rehab potential does not mean independence. It simply means potential to reach the goals the OT has set or potential for the client to make significant change.

Selecting Intervention Strategies

Occupational therapy is a dynamic process of creative problem solving with each client in each area of occupation. What is meaningful to one client may not be to another. Even a very basic task such as dressing may not seem meaningful to some clients. A person with quadriplegia who has a personal attendant, for example, may never need to dress himself, and may consider it an enormous waste of time to be required to learn to do so. However, he may be very motivated to learn to hold a mouth stick in order to engage in computer tasks for vocational retraining. Some clients will never need to balance a checkbook, while others may not be able to return to living independently without this skill. The occupational therapy practitioner asks questions like these:

- What do you want to be able to do?
- What keeps you from being able to do that?
- What are the possible options for making that happen?

The options for intervention strategies may include teaching new skills or patterns, working to increase client factors (strength, range, and endurance), or modifying the environment (context). Occupational therapy practitioners consider doing things in many different or creative ways and try to make activities meaningful and purposeful to the client.

The treatment media used by occupational therapy is also different from that used by other disciplines. OTs and OTAs often use common household objects to accomplish functional tasks. For example, the client's own clothing is a common treatment media. The clothes may be used for dressing to teach the client to don clothing or may be used for folding in order to be doing a meaningful activity while increasing standing tolerance, or for sorting colors for laundry, or for hanging in a closet to increase AROM at the shoulder. The approach would depend upon what the client will need to do in the expected discharge environment. An experienced occupational therapy practitioner can creatively find many different uses for common household objects. The same net ball that is used to wash dishes may be used for squeezing to develop grip strength, or for tactile stimulation, or for throwing to develop UE range of motion. Let us look at the intervention plan for Agnes H., which includes the goals and methods to achieve those goals.

Intervention Plan

Problem #1: Client needs min to max physical assist and verbal cues to dress self due to ↓ AROM, activity tolerance, and ability to sequence the task.

Long-term goal: Client will be able to dress with SBA and < 3 verbal cues after set-up within 2 weeks.

Short-term goals:	Interventions:
Client will don bra ① using adaptive technique within 3 days.	Teach adaptive techniques. Post picture of how to don bra correctly using adapted technique. Reinforce correct responses. Teach strengthening program for UE.
Client will don shoes and socks ① using adaptive technique and a long shoe horn within 5 days.	Provide long shoe horn and instruct client in correct use. Instruct in adaptive techniques for donning shoes and socks. Post picture of adaptive technique and long shoe horn being used to don shoes. Instruct in using affected side as a functional assist in dressing. Expand exercise program to include AROM.
Client will sequence dressing tasks correctly 3/3 tries within 1 1/2 weeks.	Verbalize steps before beginning to dress. Verbalize steps while dressing. Post list of steps for client to follow. Take rest breaks as needed for activity tolerance.

Problem #2: Client's lack of orientation to environment and inability to problem solve create safety concerns with ADL and home management.

Long-term goal: When asked, client will correctly use calendar, schedule, clock, and emergency information posted on wall within 2 weeks.

Short-term goals:	Interventions:
Client will correctly identify time, date, and situation when asked within 1 week.	Post calendar, schedule, and emergency information near clock in client's room. Instruct family, nursing staff and other therapy staff to ask client date, time, and situation several times daily and to reinforce correct responses.
Client will be able to follow a daily schedule with < 2 verbal cues within 1-2 weeks.	Post daily schedule on wall near clock. Cue client to look at schedule to determine what she should be doing at any given time.
Client will correctly problem solve responses to emergency situations with 90% accuracy within 2 weeks.	Provide situations for client to problem solve, progressing from easy to more complex. Provide telephone directory or other props as needed for problem solving.

Worksheet 12-2
Intervention Plan

Review the intervention plan for Agnes H. For each of the following criteria, determine if the necessary information is present.

Criteria	Compliance
Are specific OT interventions identified?	
Are the intervention goals and objectives measurable and realistic?	
Are the goals and objectives directly related to the client's occupational role performance?	
What is the anticipated frequency/duration of services?	
What is the discontinuation criteria or expected outcomes?	
What is the anticipated discharge location?	
What is the anticipated plan for follow-up care?	
Where will services be provided?	

Choosing Activities for Your Treatment Session

OTA students and novice clinicians often become anxious when their supervisors ask them to come up with specific treatment ideas for their clients. You might wonder how you can even begin to think of appropriate activities to target the client's needs when the client has so many issues. You might be unsure as to what to work on first or how you can achieve all the goals in such a limited time. While you will certainly collaborate with your OT supervisor, you are also expected to be able to think creatively, independently, and use your professional skills as an OTA to select appropriate treatment media or techniques. **The OT's intervention plan is your guide**. It spells out the areas to work on and the approaches to achieve those goals. For example, if a goal states, *Client will be able to ① button ½" buttons with use of buttonhook*, then your treatment session would include providing your client with a buttonhook and instructing the client how to use it. You would have the client practice buttoning and unbuttoning ½" buttons with the adaptive device. You could choose to do this on a button board or have the client practice on his shirt. A good occupational therapy activity combines working on several goals at once. If that same client also had the goal, *Client will demonstrate increased activity tolerance by standing 10 min for ADL*, you could have the client stand while practicing use of the buttonhook. Perhaps the client had a third goal, *Client will increase strength of ⓡ UE by one muscle grade in order to carry a laundry basket*. You might put a weighted cuff around the client's right wrist while the client is standing and using the buttonhook. You have now worked on three goals with one treatment activity. Let us look at another example. Suppose the OT intervention plan had the following goals:

1. *Client will demonstrate increased decision-making skills by planning a two-course meal for OT cooking group with min verbal cues within 2 weeks.*

2. *Client will demonstrate appropriate organizational skills to complete IADL within appropriate time periods within 3 weeks.*

3. *Client will demonstrate improved assertiveness by asking a peer for assistance in OT group without prompting within 2 weeks.*

Mini-Worksheet 12-3: Choosing Activities

How could you work on these goals at the same time? What would your treatment activities be? Compare your ideas with the suggestions that follow.

You might begin by having your client discuss ideas for the meal, look through a cookbook, or having him ask others in the group for ideas while he makes the final decision, all while giving verbal cues as needed. The client then can prepare the meal in the occupational therapy cooking group. You can provide the opportunity for him ask others in the group to assist with some of the steps so it can be completed within the allotted time frame. This would integrate all the goals at the same time and would be a good occupational therapy intervention. Try another scenario for the following goals in the OT's intervention plan:

1. *Student will be able to ① open all lunch containers and wrappers.*

2. *Student will spontaneously use ⓛ hand as a functional assist for bimanual classroom tasks 5/5 opportunities.*

3. *Student will attend to classroom tasks for 10-minute periods with only 1 verbal cue for redirection.*

Mini-Worksheet 12-4: Choosing Activities—More Practice

How could you work on these goals at the same time? What would your treatment activities be?

Now that you understand the initial evaluation process, you can begin to choose appropriate, realistic, and meaningful activities for your clients. Good occupational therapy activities often combine working on several goals at once to effectively achieve desired outcomes within the shortest time possible.

Chapter 13

Documenting Different
Stages of Treatment

This chapter will discuss the different types of notes written during the intervention process. These include contact notes, progress notes, reevaluation reports, transition plans, and discharge summaries. Because the OTA's primary role is to implement treatment, OTAs are most likely to write contact notes and progress notes, all under the OT's supervision. We will first look at those two types of notes in greater detail.

Contact Notes

Contact, visit, or treatment notes are used to document each visit or each individual occupational therapy session. Besides face-to-face contact with the client, these notes can also include pertinent telephone conversations or meetings with the client, family/caregiver, other professionals, or service providers. As previously discussed in Chapter 10, notes are also written stating why a scheduled session did not take place. In some situations, such as home health or acute care, contact notes are required in the health record each time a client is seen. In other circumstances, occupational therapy practitioners might keep attendance records, logs, or informal contact notes, which are used for the purpose of writing a summary of progress. The following criteria for contact notes is listed in *Guidelines for Documentation of Occupational Therapy* (AOTA 2003a):

1. Documents contacts between the client and the occupational therapist or the occupational therapy assistant. Records the types of interventions used and client's response. Includes telephone contacts, interventions, and meetings with others.

2. Suggested content with examples:

a. *Client information*—name/agency, date of birth, gender, diagnosis, precautions, and contraindications

b. *Therapy log*—date, type of contact, names/positions of persons involved, summary or significant information communicated during contacts, client attendance and participation in intervention, reason service is missed, types of interventions used, client's response, environmental or task modification, assistive or adaptive devices used or fabricated, statement of any training education or consultation provided, and the persons present

Reprinted with permission from Guidelines for Documentation of Occupational Therapy (AOTA, 2003a)

Read the following contact note from an acute care practice setting and use Worksheet 13-1 to determine how well it meets the AOTA guidelines.

XYZ Hospital
Acute Care Unit
Occupational Therapy Treatment Note

Client: John B.   **Sex**: M   **Health record #** 123456   **Date**: 4/14/06
Time: 8:30 AM   **Attending physician**: A. Smith

S: Mr. B. reports, "I feel fair today. I had a long night."

O: Client seen bedside in ICU for instruction in ADL tasks and AROM in ®̇ UE. Client nodded his head when asked if ready to sit up; required mod Ⓐ supine → sit. Upon sitting, O_2 saturation dropped to ~ 85%. Grooming, dressing and UE AROM activities not completed 2° low O_2 levels. Client required min Ⓐ to return to supine. After ~2 minutes O_2 levels returned to ~95%. Client washed face p̄ set-up in supine and nodded when asked if that felt good.

A: Client able to tolerate a little more activity today than yesterday when he did not have tolerance for supine → sit. Client also appears more motivated to attempt therapy session. Activity tolerance still limited due to O_2 saturation levels upon exertion, which limits ability to participate in self-care tasks. Client would benefit from instruction in energy conservation as well as correct positioning to ↓ exertion and ↑ activity tolerance for ADL tasks.

P: Continue skilled OT daily to ↑ activity tolerance, and Ⓘ in ADL tasks for 5 days or until discharge. Client will complete grooming EOB c̄ rest breaks as needed within 3 treatment sessions.

Bonnie B., COTA

Worksheet 13-1
Treatment, Visit, or Contact Notes

Compare the contact note for John B. to the criteria established by AOTA.

Criteria	Compliance
Is client information (name, gender, birthdate, diagnosis, precautions and/or contraindications) present?	
What is the date and time of the contact?	
What is the type of contact?	
What are the names and positions of the persons involved in the contact?	
Is there a summary of the contact or the information communicated during the contact?	
Is the client's participation in the contact (or the reason service was missed) indicated?	
Is there an indication that the task or environment was modified of that adaptive or assistive devices were used or fabricated?	
Is there an indication of any consultation/education/training and the persons involved?	

Progress Notes

Progress notes are written on a regularly scheduled basis, which might be weekly, every 2 weeks, or monthly. The facility determines the specific time frame by considering the guidelines set forth by accrediting agencies and primary payers. Progress notes provide a summary of the intervention process and record the client's progress toward goals. The *Guidelines for Documentation of Occupational Therapy* (AOTA, 2003a) list the following criteria for the content of a progress note:

---

1. Summarizes intervention process and documents client's progress toward goals achievement. Includes new data collected; modifications of treatment plan; and statement of need for continuation, discontinuation, or referral.

2. Suggested content with examples:

a. *Client information*—name/agency, date of birth, gender, diagnosis, precautions, and contraindications

b. Summary of services provided—brief statement of frequency of services and length of time services have been provided; techniques and strategies used; environmental or task modifications provided; adaptive equipment or orthotics provided; medical, educational, or other pertinent client updates; client's response to occupational therapy services; and programs or training provided to the client or caregivers

c. Current client performance—Client's progress toward the goals and client's performance in areas of occupations

d. Plan or recommendations—recommendations and rationale as well as client's input to changes or continuation of plan

Reprinted with permission from *Guidelines for Documentation of Occupational Therapy* (AOTA, 2003a).

Use the checklist on Worksheet 13-2 to compare the following progress note with the AOTA criteria.

Behavioral Health Center
Occupational Therapy Progress Note

S: *In assertion group on Tuesday 8/11/06, client talked about how her life had taken a "downward spiral" since early September, and she had become more passive and less proactive in getting her needs met, although she had not been aware of it at the time.*

O: *Client attended assertion group 2/2, communication group 1/1, and IADL group 3/5 this week. She was on time to 4/6 groups without reminders, wearing neatly pressed clothing, make-up, and an ornament in her hair. In assertion group on Thursday 8/12 she shared (without prompting) 2 stories about her usual way of dealing with retail situations. In communication group she spontaneously answered one question addressed to the group as a whole, and in IADL group she offered to assist another client with his checkbook.*

A: *Client's spontaneous actions in groups and willingness to share verbally indicate an improved mood this week. Her unprompted attendance is up this week from 2/8 to 6/8 groups. Her improved dress, hygiene, and make-up also indicate an improvement in mood from last week. Client would benefit from planning a structure for her days to prevent another "downward spiral" after discharge.*

   Goals #1: (assertion) and #2: (communication) are met as of this date.

   Goal #3: (leisure skills) is continued through discharge on 8/15/06 pending formulation of a plan.

Goal #4: (parenting skills) was discontinued on 8/10/06.

P: *Client to be seen in groups for 2 more days, with discharge anticipated on Wednesday of next
     week. IADL group will be used for preparing the structured plan for using her time. Client
     will prepare a plan including at least one planned leisure activity per day for at least 5 days out of
     7 after discharge and will discuss it with her husband and social worker by discharge on 8/15/06.*

8/13/06 Carol B., COTA
         Sharon Y., OTR/L

Worksheet 13-2
Progress Notes

Compare the behavioral health progress note to AOTA's criteria for progress notes.

Criteria	Compliance
Is client information (name, birthdate, gender, diagnosis, precautions and/or contraindications) present?	
What is the frequency of services? How long have services been provided?	
What techniques and strategies were used? Was the client or caregiver provided with programs or any training?	
Were any environmental or task modifications provided? Were any orthotic devices or adaptive equipment provided?	
What other pertinent client updates are given?	
What is the client's response to occupational therapy services?	
What progress is the client making toward her goals?	
What areas of occupation are being addressed?	
What recommendations are made and why? What is the client's input regarding continuation of the intervention plan or any changes needed?	

As you can see, contact notes and progress notes fit neatly into the SOAP format. Reevaluation reports, transition plans, and discharge summaries may also use a SOAP format but generally require more organization, analysis, intervention planning, and a broader base of knowledge. The OT is responsible for developing and documenting these documents. However, OTAs can participate in all aspects of the intervention process and can contribute to documentation at all stages under the OT's supervision (AOTA, 2004a). Therefore, we will take a brief look at reevaluations, transition plans, and discharge reports.

Reevaluation Reports

Practice settings vary regarding time frames for reevaluation. Clients might be reevaluated monthly, quarterly, or on an as-needed basis. The reevaluation is the responsibility of the OT but certain functions might be delegated to the OTA (AOTA, 2005c). According to the *Guidelines for Documentation of Occupational Therapy* (AOTA, 2003a), the reassessment report should include information about the client's condition along with a summary or update of issues, changes, or concerns that relate to the occupational profile. In addition, the tests that were given initially are readministered and the results are compared with the results of prior tests to determine the effectiveness of the treatment being provided. Revisions are then made to the goals and plans and new time lines are projected.

Hand Clinic Reevaluation Report

Client Data: **Name**: Jane P.   **DOB**: 4/01/65   **Sex**: Female   **Record #**: 12345
Primary Diagnosis: Osteoarthritis of the CMC joints bilaterally
Secondary diagnosis: None
Precautions/contraindications: None   **Referring physician**: R. Oliver, MD
Date of referral: June 27, 2006
Reason for referral: Client is 1 month post surgery (LRTI to the Ⓛ CMC joint and CTR)
Date of initial evaluation: July 5, 2006
Date of reevaluation: August 31, 2006
Funding source: University insurance

Occupational profile: Jane is a 41-year-old Caucasian female who works as an administrative assistant in the English Department at the University. She lives alone in a small two-story farmhouse 7 miles outside of town. The house is heated with wood that Jane cuts and stacks in the summer. Jane raises a large vegetable garden every year, in addition to holding both a full-time job at the University and a part-time job in a department store. She began experiencing pain in the CMC joints of both hands approximately 3 years ago. She intends to continue her present living arrangement and both of her jobs.

She was originally admitted to the outpatient hand clinic on July 5, 2006 at 1 month post surgery for hand rehabilitation following a successful LRTI and a carpal tunnel release. She is being reevaluated this date (8/31/06) to determine whether further occupational therapy services are needed.

S: Client initially reported continuous pain at a level of 3/10 and pain on overexertion of the hand at a level of 5/10, resulting in irritability and difficulty performing bilateral work and daily living tasks, as well as some tasks requiring left hand use. On this date, she reports no continuous pain and pain at a level of 1/10 when typing for more than 45 minutes without rest breaks.

Initial ability to engage in work/ADL/IADL tasks (by client report):
- Unable to use keyboard with all fingers of Ⓛ hand. Types with one finger on standard keyboard.
- Unable to grasp cylindrical objects smaller that 1½ inches (broom handle, toothpaste tube) due to ↓ AROM.
- Unable to wear watch or rings on Ⓛ hand due to swelling.
- Unable to turn door knob with Ⓛ hand to enter house when right hand is full.
- Unable to lift laundry basket and other items requiring Ⓑ UE use. Unable to lift purse or other items needed for IADL tasks c̄ with left hand.

Current ability to engage in work/ADL/IADL tasks this date (by client report):
- Able to use new ergonomic keyboard for primary work task using all fingers.
- Able to sweep the floors with a regular broom.
- Able to fold laundry using Ⓑ hands.
- Able to grasp small items needed for ADL and IADL tasks (toothpaste tube, key, lids) but not at prior level of function.

- Able to turn doorknob if door is unlocked.
- Able to hang out clothes on clothesline, including carrying basket and holding garments with left hand.

O:

Initial evaluation of client factors 7/05/06	Reassessment of client factors 8/31/06
Total active motion of the wrist: 125°	Total active motion of the wrist: 160°
Total active motion of the thumb:110°	Total active motion of the thumb: 130°
Grip strength Ⓡ 41#	Grip strength Ⓡ 40.7#
Grip strength Ⓛ 15# (31% of Ⓡ)	Grip strength Ⓛ 22.6#
Pinch not tested	Pinch not tested
Min edema	No edema

Client has been seen in outpatient hand clinic for eight 45-minute visits since admission on 7/05/06. AROM and PROM have been performed, taught to client, and home program has been modified as she progressed. Heat has been used, and the client has purchased a home paraffin unit. Electrical stimulation has been used to elicit specific motion and facilitate strengthening of the flexor pollicis longus. A strengthening program has been added to the HEP, and client is able to demonstrate all HEP exercises correctly. Client has received education on the structure and use of the hand, common features of CMC arthritis, ergonomics of the workstation, energy conservation, use of heat for pain relief, and adapted techniques for ADL activities. Client reports understanding the education, and has been given written material covering the same content.

A: Increase in grip strength of 7# shows good progress in strength needed to perform functional tasks. Thumb AROM is now WFL, and wrist AROM is increased 35° to 80% of average, allowing client to perform most work and ADL tasks Ⓘ in ways that do not damage the joint. Change to an ergonomic keyboard and understanding and correct self-administration of HEP indicate good potential to continue improvement without continued occupational therapy services.

P: Client to call hand clinic if questions arise, and follow the home program of heat, exercise, and adapted techniques. Results of reevaluation indicate no further need for occupational therapy services unless new problems arise.

Brad E., OTR/L, CHT

Worksheet 13-3
Reevaluation Reports

Review the hand clinic reevaluation report and determine if the necessary information is present.

Criteria	Compliance
Is there any new information about the client's medical condition or occupational profile?	
What was the purpose of the reevaluation?	
What assessments were used initially? What assessments are used now?	
How do the results compare with the previous evaluation results?	
What occupational changes are evident? In what ways has the client made progress?	
Are there areas of occupation that are still problematic?	
What changes in occupational therapy treatment, goals, or referrals will be made as a result of the reevaluation?	

Transition Plans

A transition plan is developed and written whenever a client transfers within a service delivery system from one setting to another (AOTA, 2003a). This is the responsibility of the OT but, as with other stages of treatment, the OTA can contribute to this process (AOTA, 2005c). The purpose of the transition plan is to provide client information to the new service providers to prevent any interruption in care. According to the *Guidelines for Documentation of Occupational Therapy* (AOTA, 2003a), a transition plan summarizes the client's current occupational status, specifies what service setting the client is leaving, what setting the client is entering, and states how and when the transition will occur. It also lists what follow-up or recommended services would benefit the client such as continued therapy, specific equipment, or necessary modifications.

XYZ Early Intervention Program
Occupational Therapy Department
Transition Plan

Name: Julie M.   **Date of birth**: 4/29/03   **Gender**: Female   **Record #**: 87654
Date of plan: April 11, 2006   **Expected Transition Date**: May, 2006
Precautions/contraindications: Seizure disorder

Occupational history: Julie experienced head and orthopedic injuries following a MVA at 9 days of age. Since that time she has had multiple cranial, hip, and leg surgeries. She is currently under the management of a neurologist as well as an orthopedist. The mother carries out a home program daily that is designed to stimulate development.

S: The mother reports that although Julie's seizures, multiple surgeries, and illnesses have slowed her development, the family is hopeful that Julie will progress more rapidly through her developmental milestones now that the surgeries are finished and the seizures are under control.

O: Child received her first occupational therapy screening in the hospital 1 week post injury. She received formal developmental assessments at 2, 4, 6, 12 and 24 months of age. Parents were given home program following the initial formal assessment. Regular occupational therapy treatment sessions were started at 12 months of age and have continued to this date. Child has been seen twice weekly in her home and monthly in the Birth-to-Three clinic. She is now eligible, due to her age, for preschool services.
Current occupational performance: Current problems being treated in occupational therapy include visual regard and visually directed reach, midline orientation, postural symmetry, and motor overflow. Current goals for Julie include functional reach, grasp and release, rolling, and ability to sustain antigravity positions for ADL and developmental play activities.

A: At 3 years of age, Julie is at about a 4-month level of development. Although the mother provides a stimulating environment, Julie would benefit from continuation of regular occupational therapy, physical therapy, and speech therapy services to facilitate her continued progress through the developmental sequence.

P: Julie will receive her first preschool service evaluation next month in May of 2006. Parents have been given a home program, which has been updated as child has progressed in treatment. Home program will continue through the transition to preschool services.

Worksheet 13-4
Transition Plan

Review the transition plan for Julie and determine if the necessary information is present according to the AOTA guidelines.

Criteria	Compliance
What is the client's occupational performance at this time?	
What is the current setting?	
What will the new setting be?	
What is the reason for the transition?	
When will the transition occur?	
What activities will occur throughout the transition?	
What recommendations are made for occupational therapy services in the new setting?	
What other recommendations, equipment, or follow-up are indicated in this plan?	

Table 13-1.
Reasons for Discharge

- Occupational therapy outcomes were met.
- Client discharged from facility or agency.
- No further occupational therapy is necessary.
- Duplication of services.
- Client not making progress.
- Client became ill/was hospitalized.
- MD discontinued therapy.
- Reimbursement issues/managed care.
- Client requires more specialized services than can be provided at this facility.
- Client noncompliant or refusing therapy.
- Poor attendance.
- Client expired.
- Client moved.
- Client decided to receive services elsewhere.

Discharge Summaries

A discharge summary (also called a "discontinuation report") provides a synopsis of the changes or progress regarding the client's ability to engage in occupation. These reports also include recommendations for referral or follow-up care if needed. Discharge reports are the responsibility of the OT but the therapist can delegate parts of this process to the OTA as appropriate (AOTA, 2005c). Discharge notes often follow a specific format. Content should include the date and purpose of the referral, a summary of the client's condition, comparison of initial evaluation findings to status at time of discharge, and the course of treatment such as types of interventions/programs, physical agent modalities, splints, assistive devices, modifications, and client/caregiver education. Discharge reports also include a summary of progress and outcomes relating to occupational performance, along with recommendations for follow-up care (AOTA, 2003a). Recommendations may include continued therapy, home exercise programs, specific equipment, necessary modifications, or recommended support groups or community services. Some settings or third party payers require that the number of occupational therapy sessions provided also be listed. Discharge summaries may be done as a SOAP or narrative format, or the facility may have a particular form that is used. Some facilities use the same or similar form for evaluation, reevaluation and discharge, making it easier to prepare the discontinuation report.

There are many reasons that an OT client is discharged or treatment is discontinued. It is important for the discharge report to indicate the circumstances or reasons for discharge. Table 13-1 lists possible reasons for discontinuing occupational therapy.

The discontinuation note we will be evaluating in Worksheet 13-5 is written in a SOAP format, and then presented again as it might be written on a facility form, so that you can see it done both ways.

XYZ Rehabilitation Center
Occupational Therapy Department
Discharge Summary

Name: Sally J.   **Record #:** 123456   **DOB**: 11/10/32
Date: 10/19/06   **Time**: 3:00 PM   **Gender**: F

S: Client reports that she is very pleased with the outcome of her occupational therapy treatment, and with her ability to take care of herself at home. She reports no steps to the front entrance of a one-story home, and no architectural barriers inside the house. She reports that she owns the following adaptive equipment already: wheeled walker, reacher, dressing stick, sock aid, long shoe horn, tub bench, raised toilet seat, and grab bars around the toilet and in the tub.

O: Client seen bedside and in clinic area 20/20 sessions from SOC on 9/25/06.

ADL status on 9/25/06	ADL status on 10/19/06
Mod Ⓐ in transfers.	SBA in transfers
Mod Ⓐ in toileting.	Ⓘ in toileting.
Mod Ⓐ in feeding.	SBA in feeding after set-up.
Mod Ⓐ in dressing.	Dressing from arm chair requires set up only, but SBA for standing and pulling pants up over hips.
Max Ⓐ for safety in bathing.	SBA in bathing with min Ⓐ w/c ↔ shower using tub bench.

Client education in adaptive techniques and HEP were discussed with client and client demonstrated ability to perform correctly. Home modifications discussed with client and caregiver.

A: Client has made good progress in self-care activities and shown by differences in admitting and discharge abilities. Since caregiver is available to provide SBA needed for safety in ADL tasks, all treatment goals have been met, and client is ready for discontinuation of occupational therapy services.

P: Client to continue home exercise program. Adaptive equipment recommended: walker basket and reacher holder for walker. Client and caregiver to decide how to implement home modifications. Client to continue outpatient physical therapy. No direct occupational therapy services recommended at this time.

Now let us consider the same discharge note, written on a form provided by the rehabilitation facility.

XYZ Rehabilitation Center
Occupational Therapy Department
Discharge Note

Name: Sally J.   **Record #:** 123456   **DOB**: 11/10/32
Date: 10/19/06   **Time**: 3:00 PM   **Gender**: F

Course of Rehabilitation:
Client seen 20/20 sessions from SOC on 9/25/06. Skilled instruction in adaptive techniques for ADL provided. Client progress was good and she met all tx. goals. Client now requires SBA in all transfers, lower body ADL, upper body ADL, grooming/hygiene. She is Ⓘ in toileting. Client also requires SBA in feeding after set-up. Dressing from arm chair with wheeled walker, set-up only but SBA for standing and to pull pants up over hips. Bathing is SBA with min Ⓐ w/c ↔ shower using tub bench.

Client Education:
Recommendations for additional adaptive equipment and modifications to home discussed with client and caregiver. Client and caregiver were instructed in home exercise program of Theraband, free weights, wands, and other activities to choose from for Ⓑ UE strengthening. HEP discussed with client and client demonstrated ability to perform exercises correctly.

Discharge Recommendations/Referrals:
Discharge with home caregiver. Continue home exercise program. Adaptive equipment recommended: walker basket and reacher holder for walker. Client already has wheeled walker, reacher, dressing stick, sock aid, long shoehorn, and functional bathroom equipment and has demonstrated ability to use these correctly and safely. Client will be seen in outpatient PT. No direct OT services are recommended at this time.

Paul H., OTR/L

Worksheet 13-5
Discharge Summary

Do the discharge summaries for Sally J. include all the pertinent information? Does one format provide information in a better way?

Criteria	Compliance
Is information present about the client's medical condition? How has the condition changed?	
What was the initial date of OT service? What was the end date of OT service? Are the number of intervention sessions listed?	
What types of interventions were provided? What was the client's progress toward goals?	
What was the client's beginning and ending status regarding ability to engage in occupations?	
Was the client satisfied with outcomes?	
What recommendations or follow-up are listed? How well do they pertain to the future needs of the client?	

You have learned the basic criteria for different types of occupational therapy documentation. The next chapter will discuss documentation in different practice settings so you can understand the requirements in various areas of clinical practice.

Chapter 14

Documentation in Different Practice Settings

This chapter will look at documentation for different practice settings, each of which has some requirements specific to the setting or the primary source of payment. Documentation for these situations is different in some ways from the examples you have learned so far.

Documentation in Mental Health

If you go from a job in a rehabilitation center to one in a mental health setting, you might think that nothing you have learned about documentation applies. Some mental health issues (such as suicide risk or past sexual abuse) may not conform very neatly into the *Framework* (Holmquist, 2004) and the language used in documentation may appear more subjective and general than what you have learned thus far. Also, a multidisciplinary approach is used in mental health settings to establish problems, goals, and interventions. Occupational therapy is often regarded as part of a broader treatment service designated as adjunctive therapy, expressive therapy, or activity therapy; disciplines that fall under this umbrella include therapeutic recreation specialists, music therapists, art therapists, and dance therapists. Professional roles often overlap and there is a blurring of professional identities. Intervention is provided in groups or as part of a therapeutic environment or milieu. Reimbursement may not be discipline specific and therapy services may be included in the comprehensive room rate for the facility.

Occupational therapy practitioners have traditionally considered the holistic needs of those who receive our services. We look at the physical, cognitive, social, and emotional factors that affect role performance and quality of life. Occupational therapy practitioners intervene to promote psychosocial well-being and to facilitate engagement in desired life activities across all practice areas. Our clients in mental health settings have significant psychosocial problems that create serious disruptions in their abilities to take part in meaningful occupations. Occupational therapy practitioners in this practice area have a "toolbox" of psychosocial interventions that are a viable and fundamental component of occupational therapy practice.

Evaluation Reports and Intervention Plans

Initial evaluation reports may be performed by the OT, with contributions from the OTA. However, evaluation reports are often, instead, a collaborative effort involving all the disciplines included in activity therapy, thereby losing some of the individual professional identity of occupational therapy. Due to reimbursement issues, facilities often must bundle therapy into the room rate rather than billing individual therapies separately. Having an integrated "activities" or adjunctive therapy department is usually more cost-effective than having a separate occupational therapy department. Even so, occupational therapy practitioners should consider an occupational profile essential in order to plan appropriate and effective interventions as the *Framework* indicates (AOTA, 2002). Mental illness and chemical dependency impact quality of life and ability to engage in meaningful occupations. The OT, with assistance from the OTA, looks at the areas of occupation that are disrupted by the client's condition, the dysfunctional behaviors manifested by the illness (and psychotropic medication side effects), the influencing contextual factors, available supports, and the client's goals. The occupational therapy practitioners use this information to contribute to the treatment team's multidisciplinary problem list and intervention plan.

The *therapeutic milieu*, or the setting's total environment, is often considered essential in caring for clients who have mental illnesses. Ideally, each discipline assesses the client's needs and strengths and then the team meets to formulate and prioritize a list of the client's problems. Problems in a mental health practice setting are traditionally divided into two parts. First, the problem itself is stated in one or two words, such as "chemical dependence," "noncompliant behavior," or "suicide risk." Next, a description of the behavioral manifestations indicates the areas of occupation and underlying limiting factors involved.

Problem: Suicide risk

Behavioral manifestations: During the week prior to admission, the client verbalized suicidal ideation, stating that life was no longer worth living. On the day of admission he purchased a handgun.

Problem: Chemical dependence

Behavioral manifestations: Mark has been using alcohol since age 12 with increasing frequency over the last year, and also admits to using cocaine, "crystal", opium, and marijuana, resulting in a failed marriage, loss of two jobs, and involvement with the criminal justice system.

Problem: Noncompliant behavior

Behavioral manifestations: Client disobeys foster parents by running away, refusing to follow rules or requests, and engaging in sexual activity, resulting in six foster home placements in the past 4 years.

From this problem list, each individual discipline suggests goals, objectives, and treatment interventions appropriate to that discipline. In community mental health settings, occupational therapy goals can be related more easily and clearly to areas of occupational engagement. An individualized treatment plan (ITP) is developed, which is a contract for change between the client and the treatment team. Major concerns or problems identified in the evaluation are documented on the ITP and each discipline's goals, objectives, and interventions are written into one comprehensive plan. The client collaborates in the intervention process, and signs the treatment plan to demonstrate agreement with it. Similar types of plans are developed by teams in schools and rehabilitation settings but mental health plans differ in that all clinicians work toward the same goals through different interventions. At some facilities, goals and objectives are selected from computer programs or provided on preprinted sheets for the problems most commonly treated, as illustrated later in this chapter. Because of short length of stay and the multidisciplinary nature of the intervention plan, discharge goals may not be broken down into short-term goals. A client may even be discharged before a comprehensive treatment plan can be formalized.

In order for multidisciplinary treatment plans to be successful, the client (and family, if they are a part of the client's present life) must be actively involved. Each member of the treatment team must be willing to cooperate in a coordinated effort to effect change. In addition, the plan must be periodically reviewed to assess its effectiveness and to change or modify any interventions that have not been effective.

Intervention Strategies

OTs and OTAs use communication techniques and therapeutic use of self as part of the occupational therapy process to establish client relationships, identify meaningful occupations, and determine barriers to occupational performance (Kannenberg and Greene, 2003). OTs and OTAs use a variety of interventions in mental health to promote empowerment, facilitate a positive self-concept, and enable personal change. Interventions are directed toward helping the client develop or remediate specific life skills for occupational roles within the home, community, and other contexts. Occupational therapy practitioners may provide specific instruction and practice in adaptive mechanisms/techniques, symptom/behavior management, temporal organization, assertiveness training, strategies for coping with stress and anger, communication/interaction skills, and task behaviors.

Interventions may be specific to occupational therapy, or may be broader and applicable to activity therapy. Often, the choice of interventions depends largely upon what treatment groups are being provided by the facility. Intervention strategies are implemented within the groups, creating an interesting challenge for the OTA to address each client's particular needs at the same time. For example, most clients may attend communication groups or craft/activity groups, but within those groups, you will customize the way you choose to increase communication skills or improve task behaviors for each individual client. With a little experience, you will learn to individualize goals effectively for each participant, while still providing for the needs of the group as a whole.

When planning intervention strategies, the treatment team considers the client's assets (intelligence, good verbal skills, etc.) as important tools that the client will use in overcoming her problems. A "strength" in this context is an ability, a skill, or an interest that the client has used in the past or has the potential for using. Assets can include such things as the client's interests (enjoys playing music, gardening, knitting), abilities (writes well, accepts personal responsibility, is well organized), relationship skills (has a good relationship with her adult daughter), and social support systems (AA group, minister keeps in contact). Assets may also be past abilities that the treatment team wants to encourage as treatment progresses (Carol was physically active before she became ill). Some interests (enjoys going to bars or casinos on weekends) may not be assets if they contribute to maladaptive behavior.

Ideally, occupational therapy documentation in psychosocial programs should be objective, measurable, realistic, and reflective of the occupation base of our profession. This means that your documentation must center on the client's occupational profile and the client's ability to engage in necessary and valued life activities.

Contact and Progress Notes

The use of contact and progress notes may vary by facility. If a client with a mental health diagnosis is seen in home health, the Medicare standards for home health, which require treatment notes for each visit, apply. In a situation where progress notes rather than treatment notes are used, the occupational therapy practitioner keeps a log of attendance and makes notes to himself about participation and behaviors that show progress each day. These personal notations are then compiled into a progress note in the health record at regular intervals.

When you begin thinking in the language of mental health, terms like "brightened affect," "less delusional," "improved mood," or "increased self-esteem" begin to enter your vocabulary, and you may be tempted to write in less objective and measurable terms. However, there are definite observable behaviors (also called behavioral justifications) that can help you determine weaknesses or strengths such as the client's affect is brighter or his mood is improved. Perhaps you are seeing her begin to apply make-up, smile more frequently, initiate conversation more often, or respond to your "good morning" by making eye contact. Perhaps the client needs less time to get up and dress in the morning, is more easily persuaded to attend OT, or is able to select and carefully complete a craft project without verbal prompting. All these indicators are measurable, and it is very helpful to the treatment team if you are able to report your skilled observations in measurable and behavioral terms.

Managed care, along with the trend toward role diffusion, is making it more difficult to document occupational therapy as a service that offers good value for the dollars spent in mental health care. You, as an OTA, need to focus on documenting functional changes that are cost-effective and meaningful to both the payer and to the consumer. Individuals with serious mental illness and chemical dependency often have myriad factors that hinder their ability to engage in meaningful occupation. OTs and OTAs working in mental health settings need to communicate clearly how our unique services impact the client's ability to achieve "successful, meaningful, and lasting functional outcomes" (Kannenberg and Greene, p. CE-1, 2003).

Critical Care Pathways in Mental Health

As length of stay has becomes shorter for psychiatric diagnoses, some mental health settings have started using critical care pathways and computer generated intervention plans for the most common problems seen in that setting. These methods save time and can be customized to the client by adding desired outcomes and treatment interventions tailored to the individual's needs. Critical care pathways in mental health are multidisciplinary and are conceptually the same as those in rehabilitation. The plan for the client's care is preplanned for each day and for each discipline. This makes the most efficient use of staff time during the client's short length of stay, while still making sure the client's needs are met.

Computer Generated Plans

In an electronic "mix-and-match" program, the computer provides prompts from which the team or the individual clinician selects the problem statements, goals, objectives, and treatment interventions that will be used for the individual consumer. Usually the problems are expressed briefly in these prepackaged treatment planning sheets, such as depressed mood, drug abuse, or suicide risk. Then the client's specific behavioral manifestations are written in.

The treatment team then chooses the client's goals from a menu of long-term goals, or **outcomes**, such as these:

- *Client will report the absence of suicidal ideation.*

    OR

- *Client will identify three new coping strategies to use when he feels the urge to use drugs.*

During the client's hospitalization, all members of the interdisciplinary treatment team work on the selected goals. On a computer generated form, there is also a list of potential interventions that would also be selected and addressed by the treatment team. Interventions on this menu might include such strategies as the following:

- Evaluate the client.
- Encourage client to express emotions.
- Teach new coping skills.
- Encourage the client to verbalize alternatives to previous coping strategies.
- Assist the client to develop a discharge plan that will prevent recurrence.

Appropriate interventions are chosen for use with each client and each discipline implements the interventions in its own way. Social work adapts interventions to individual and group therapy, nursing implements the interventions on the unit, whereas occupational therapy will implement the interventions in groups and in activities relating to occupational performance. In regard to the five intervention strategies listed above, the OTA might do the following:

- Assist the OT in data collection for the occupational profile.
- Assist the OT in determining specific problems in each area of occupation.
- Use occupational therapy media to encourage the client to express emotions.
- Use occupational therapy groups to teach new coping skills and to help the client to find alternatives to strategies that have not worked well in the past.
- Provide feedback to the OT and client regarding task behaviors and performance skills as they relate to occupational performance.
- Help the client make a plan for any areas of occupation that were part of the previous problem.

In order to implement the multidisciplinary interventions, sheets are provided for each of the common goals. The interventions are individualized to the client by stating behavioral manifestations of the problem and by adding and deleting outcomes and/or interventions. The sheets also list the responsible staff member. This chapter includes an example of a prepackaged treatment planning sheet for alcohol dependence. It is provided only as a representation of what might be seen in clinical practice. Each setting will have its own protocols, but this will give you an idea of how a problem might be handled.

Let us consider another example—a female client admitted to a psychiatric unit following a suicide attempt. If the treatment team were using a computer generated plan for this client, the first step would be to go to the computer and pull up some multidisciplinary treatment planning sheets. Some of the choices might be:

- Suicide attempt
- Anger
- Poor self-esteem

On each sheet there would be a place to identify the client's behavior in relation to the problem.

Problem: Suicide attempt

Behavioral manifestations: During 2 days prior to admission, the client verbalized suicidal ideation, stating that her life was no longer worth living. On the day of admission, she took an overdose of sleeping pills and was brought to the ER by ambulance.

Problem: Anger

Behavioral Manifestations: For the past 6 months, client has been fighting with her husband resulting in marital separation, physical destruction of household objects, and high levels of stress.

Problem: Poor self-esteem

Behavioral Manifestations: For the past month, client has shown diminished interest in her appearance, resulting in an unkempt look at home and work. She has been verbalizing self-deprecating statements regarding her looks, self-worth, and future plans.

Next follows a list of interventions commonly used for that problem, starting with evaluation and ending with discharge planning. Interventions on the list that do not apply to this client would be deleted, and any additional interventions unique to this client would be written in. The list of interventions would include some similar interventions as the previous example such as, *"Encourage client to express emotions"* and *"Teach new coping skills,"* and other interventions would be added for this particular situation such as *"Encourage positive self-concept."* The groups provided by the facility would be listed as interventions, and the OT and OTA would plan for ways to make the daily occupational therapy groups meet the client's needs. There would be a list of desired outcomes for each of the clients' identified problems, with a place to add outcomes specific to the situation.

Behavioral Health Multidisciplinary Treatment Plan

Client Name: **Record #**
Problem #:   **Problem name:** Alcohol Dependence
Date Identified: **Behavioral manifestations:**

Desired Outcomes	Target Date:	Date achieved:
1. Client will verbally acknowledge that alcohol use has been a problem and will state intent to abstain from alcohol use.		
2. Client will have developed at least three new ways to manage stress and will have demonstrated use of these.		
3. Client will have an aftercare plan in place.		
4. Client will have established a 5-day period of sobriety and of attending AA meetings daily.		
5.		
6.		

Treatment Interventions	Staff Responsible
1. Evaluation of the client's alcohol intake and use patterns.	
2. Provide individual, group, and family therapy.	
3. Education re: the disease model of chemical dependency.	
4. Provide opportunities to express feelings.	
5. Teach coping skills.	
6. Assist client to restructure environmental situations.	
7. Evaluate and teach relationship skills.	
8. Facilitate peer confrontation and feedback.	
9. Introduce social/leisure activities that do not include alcohol.	
10.	
11.	

I agree with this plan

_____
Client's signature

Documentation in School Based Practice

Occupational therapy practitioners working in the public school system use concepts and language that are unique to that setting. Therefore, documentation in school settings is different from the notes occupational therapy practitioners might write in other practice areas. The children in your school caseload will each have an **intervention plan** called an **Individualized Education Program** (IEP). This IEP consists of problems, goals, and interventions that are **educationally based**; that is, focused on behaviors and skills the student needs to be successful in school. The IEP is a multidisciplinary plan that is established at an annual meeting for each child classified as needing special services. The plan is compiled by therapists, teachers, and parents, plus any other appropriate professionals involved with the child (such as a psychologist, blind mobility specialist, sign language interpreter, social worker, or special educator).

The OT is responsible for directing the occupational therapy evaluation, establishing the occupational therapy goals or objectives for the IEP, and implementing or overseeing occupational therapy treatment. The OTA will provide feedback throughout this process and will implement delegated assessments and interventions. The IEP is a collaborative effort. Based on each discipline's assessment, the IEP details the current educational status, problems, goals, and interventions for the child in all areas (including occupational therapy) for the current school year. The treatment principles and concepts for the entire team are basically the same. The language, however, is different for each discipline and that is very important for establishing each professional's role.

Functional problem statements are exclusively problems of engaging in occupation in the educational setting, even though the child may have many deficits in other areas of life. These educational problems might address:

- Classroom behaviors and skills (attention to task, handwriting, scissors use, copying from blackboard, etc.)
- Academic performance
- Personal and toilet hygiene (combing hair, washing hands, feminine hygiene, managing clothing)
- Dressing (putting on coat or boots, changing for gym)
- Feeding (opening lunch containers/wrappers, handling finger foods, utensils, or tray)
- Ability to participate in extracurricular activities (drama, music, clubs, sports)
- Ability to manage the activity demands for various school contexts (cafeteria, gym, recess, locker room)
- Ability to navigate around the school (mobility, managing backpack, locker use)
- Ability to appropriately relate to staff and peers

Goal statements are normally written for the duration of the school year, rather than using a time line for each goal. In this setting, goals for the school year are called *objectives*. Sometimes the format is slightly different, with a *criteria* added to make the goal specific. These criteria can include specific academic standards (grade level, district, or state), developmental milestones, professional judgment, peer performance, and parent or teacher expected outcomes (Clark, 2005). The child may be assessed quarterly to grade or determine progress toward meeting the established benchmarks. In a school setting, it is very important to set goals for specific educational components rather than underlying factors. Goals should be clearly written and defined so that the child's specific expected behavior or criterion can be observed and measured by others (Clark, 2005). Interventions are specific to the educational setting as well, even though the child may also need treatment for problems in other areas of occupation.

IEPs can be quite lengthy. The one provided in this chapter has been condensed from its original 26 pages to show aspects that are representative or most pertinent to occupational therapy.

Individualized Education Program

Student: Truman T.   **Date of birth:** 9/17/93   **Parents**: Linda and Ellis T.
Teacher: Mary Ellen W.   **Case manager**: Sharon Y.   **IEP conference date**: 5/23/06
Annual review date: 5/23/07 **Duration of services**: 1 year   **Initial placement date**: 9/27/99
Service model: Regular education: 100 minutes,   initiated 5/24/05   ending 5/24/06
                          Special education: 1550 minutes   initiated 5/24/05   ending 5/24/06
Related services: Occupational therapy, physical therapy, adaptive PE, special transportation
Placement: Self-contained classroom
Assistive devices: Glasses   **Physical education**: Adaptive PE
Special transition services needed: Instruction, related services, daily living skills
Specialized materials: Easel, bookstand for academic and fine motor activities, enlarged monitor for computer, pencil grip.
Notification of progress: Parents will be given a copy of the goals and progress 4 times per year with the report card.

Present level of performance: Truman has been diagnosed with cerebral palsy (quadriplegic), developmental delays, and visual difficulties. He wears glasses and needs written work enlarged. He has a history of ear infections and has bilateral tubes in place. Truman displays low muscle tone, with compensatory fluctuating increased tone upon movement. Fine motor skills include spasticity noted in both arms on passive range of motion. Grip strength has improved, but bilateral tasks remain difficult due to poor lateral trunk control. He requires minimal to moderate assistance to hold his arms in different positions simultaneously. He requires moderate assistance to use scissors. His speech and language skills are commensurate with his intellectual functioning, in the mentally handicapped range of abilities. The WISC II suggests that his general information and verbal reasoning skills are at a 6 year age level. Non-verbal abilities are at about the same level. Truman shows difficulty with visual-spatial abilities, visual-motor integration, gross-motor production, and visual-perceptual processing. Vocabulary is low. He has a relative strength in short term auditory memory and ability to sequence small bits of information. His ability to perceive patterns and relations is impaired, as is his neuropsychological processing of tactile stimuli. His adaptive behavior is below average. Current level of functioning is the 1.0 - 1.5 grade level. Reading comprehension and spelling ability are age equivalent 6-0, with math computation at an age level of 7-0. Adaptive functioning suggests an age equivalent of approximately 5-0 years. He is able to use a telephone in an emergency, look both ways before crossing the street, and get a drink of water from a tap unassisted. Progress has been made in adaptive functioning, but significant deficits remain in regard to toileting, dressing, functional mobility, and food preparation skills. No significant behavioral difficulties exist either at school or at home. Truman has limited interactions with peers, and limited participation in the regular classroom. He attends technology lab twice a week with a student aide. He works best on a 1-1 basis for 15-20 minute intervals in a situation where auditory distractions are limited.

Annual Goal #1: Truman will show school /homework responsibilities
Implementer: Special Education Teacher
Evaluation procedure: Observation
Short-term objective #1: Truman will be responsible for homework in different areas of study at least 2 times weekly.
Short-term objective #2: Truman will be responsible for taking notebook home and returning it the following day. Homework assignments consisting of spelling words, reading and math sheets, counting change, and telling time. Worksheets will be listed in this book.

Annual Goal #2: Truman will improve skills in adaptive physical education
Implementer: Adaptive PE teacher/paraprofessional
Short-term objective: Truman will sit up.
Evaluation procedure: Observation
Criteria: Without being reminded for 1/2 hour

Annual goal #4: Truman will use computers in the classroom and computer lab.
Implementer: Special Education teacher/paraprofessionals

Short term objective: Truman will use computers with assistance
Evaluation procedure: Observation   **Criteria**: 80% accuracy

Annual goal #5: Truman will improve math skill.
Implementer: Special Education Teacher
Objective #1: Given a clock dial, Truman will say the time to the 5-minute interval
Evaluation procedure: Daily work   **Criteria**: 80% accuracy 3 of 4 tracking days

Annual goal #6: Improve fine motor skills for greater success with classroom related activities
Implementer: Occupational Therapist
Short-term objective #1: Truman will cut 8" using adaptive scissors with minimal assistance to adjust grasp and paper position.
Evaluation Procedure: Daily work   **Criteria**: 75% accuracy
Short-term objective #2: Truman will type 10 spelling words on adaptive computer keyboard using isolated index finger movements.
Evaluation Procedure: Daily work   **Criteria**: No more than 2 errors

Annual Goal #7: Increase visual motor skills for greater success in academic work
Implementer: Occupational Therapist
Short-term objective: Truman will demonstrate good attention to task and visual motor skills in order to sort 15 small items.
Evaluation procedure: Observation   **Criteria**: Within 90 seconds with minimal verbal cues and 75% accuracy

Annual Goal #8: Truman will exhibit increased functional motor skills in the school environment.
Implementer: Physical Therapist
Short-term objective: Sitting on a box, Truman will lean forward and sit upright picking up objects from the floor
Evaluation procedure: Observation   **Criteria**: 8 times with 50% assistance from therapist after 10 consecutive sessions

Least restrictive environment: Self-contained special education classroom
Related services: Occupational therapy, physical therapy, transportation, assistive technology, language therapy
Will student be receiving services in school closest to home? X yes _ no
IEP services that cannot be provided in the regular classroom: Math, reading, written expression, listening comprehension, language, physical therapy, occupational therapy, transition
<u>**Factors for consideration of removal**</u>:

1. **Nature and severity of the disability**

   Difficulty performing activity of daily living at an age-appropriate level

   Receptive/expressive language skills interfere with communication

   Easily distracted/frequently off task

2. **Diverse learning style of the student**:

   Requires highly structured small-group setting

   Lacks social/behavioral skills for participation in regular classroom

   Requires exposure to experiences not available in regular classroom

   Individualized instruction

   Increased drill/practice to master skills

   Immediate corrective feedback

   Additional time to complete task

   Positive rewards

3. **Inability to engage appropriately with other students**:

Requires inordinate amount of teacher time

Learning styles cannot be addressed in regular classroom

Expressive language skills inadequate for classroom participation

Receptive language skills interfere with academic progress

Occupational Therapy Evaluation/Progress Report

This 13-year-old male has received occupational therapy services throughout his school years with intervention most recently three times weekly for 45-minute sessions to work on improving fine motor and visual motor skills. Truman lives with his parents, who are very supportive, active in his care, and motivated to see him succeed to his highest potential. He has many adaptations in his home to promote independence and assist caregivers.

Truman presents as friendly and kind, and wanting to please. He apologizes when he is unable to complete what is asked of him, although at times he will complain of being too tired to complete a task. He is very social and gets along with both peers and adults. Due to his cognitive limitations, standard testing would not give valid results. For this reason, observation of functioning has been used.

Fine Motor

Low muscle tone with moderate spasticity noted Ⓑ upon PROM. Elbows are contracted by calcium deposits to -30° Ⓡ and -40° Ⓛ. Truman is Ⓡ hand dominant. Grip strength Ⓡ is from 15-20# and Ⓛ from 8-16# in the past year. Truman has difficulty with Ⓑ tasks due to lateral trunk instability, which requires use of one hand to stabilize himself. He has a hypersensitive startle reflex, which activates when he feels like he is losing his balance. He has been working on disassociating arms so that he can use one for movement while the other is doing a different movement, and requires moderate assistance to do this. He is able to open a soda can after the seal has been broken with extra time given. He requires verbal reminders 75% of the time to use his Ⓛ arm to stabilize an object with one hand while manipulating it with the other. He requires moderate assist for scissors use and requires assistance to stabilize the paper. His arms become stiffened as he recruits all his muscle fibers to hold on to scissors and paper. Despite this, he has made great gains in scissors use over the past year.

Visual Motor/Visual Perception

Truman has severe visual problems and needs adaptive equipment to compensate for his visual deficits, including a large screen monitor and adaptive keyboard with the letters in alphabetical order. For future use, an adapted keyboard with enlarged letters in the regular order is recommended. He is able to use the mouse to move coins on the screen into a narrow slot with 75% accuracy.

Truman has a poor ability to track objects and poor ocular motor control. It is hard to tell what he can see, because he often guesses at responses. He is able to find objects in the classroom and to maneuver his wheelchair around obstacles. He has demonstrated great gains in visual motor paper and pencil skills, progressing from the inability to draw vertical and horizontal lines to the ability to copy circles, squares, and triangles with moderate assistance and dot-to-dot guides. Adaptive equipment (vertical slant board and enlarged writing utensils) are needed for writing.

Gross Motor

Overall low tone with compensatory fluctuating increased tone upon movement. Specific exercises are performed daily as a part of adaptive PE.

Sensory Integration

No sensory defensiveness or unusual sensory behaviors.

Self-Help

- Functional mobility: Able to wheel his chair within school environment with extra time.
- Eating: He generally chooses finger foods but has demonstrated ability to use utensils with built-up handles.
- Toileting, Dressing (coat), Wheelchair Positioning: Requires moderate assistance for these tasks. He is very private with his toileting and prefers males to assist him. He often slides forward in his wheelchair and has difficulty sitting upright and righting himself once he has leaned to the side. He would benefit from a wheelchair back that provides some lateral support and a cushion that will decrease the slide forward.

Summary

Truman has made great gains in fine motor strength and visual motor skills over the past year. Harrington rod placement greatly increased his ability to interact within the school environment. He seems motivated to succeed. Strengths include his supportive family, his motivation, his general good health, and emotional stability. Areas of concern continue to be his muscle weakness with compensatory abnormal movement patterns and visual motor/visual perceptual difficulties. If daily strengthening continues to be provided by school staff, Truman would benefit from occupational therapy at a decreased rate to focus on monitoring and training staff to assist him with exercise, visual motor and bilateral coordination tasks.

Recommendations

Continue occupational therapy services twice weekly for 45-minute sessions to work on areas of concern listed above. Continue use of adaptive equipment listed above. Begin transitional planning for skills necessary after high school.

Linda E., OTR/L

Skilled Nursing Facilities and Long-Term Care

Many clients who receive subacute rehabilitation services in skilled nursing facilities are covered by Medicare. Therefore, occupational therapy documentation must reflect the need for skilled services such as the potential for functional change, to address safety concerns, or to prevent secondary medical complications. Intervention will address skills needed for the client to return home or to improve functional performance skills for other contexts. This may include improving activity tolerance, safe functional mobility, or ADL. Occupational therapy intervention may also include recommending, fabricating, or modifying adaptive equipment, splints, positioning devices, or wheelchairs. Clients sometimes participate in occupational therapy groups that address particular occupational performance skills or client factors such as a cooking group or an UE exercise group. Clients who are not considered subacute may also receive occupational therapy services if skilled occupational therapy is warranted. In these cases, occupational therapy will address particular problem areas identified in the care plan and therapy is usually only indicated for a short-term basis.

When a client is first admitted to a skilled nursing facility, a multidisciplinary evaluation called the Minimum Data Set (MDS) is used to determine the level of care needed. The MDS is an assessment tool and quality measure that considers all aspects of the client such as mood, behavior, mobility, ADL status, bowel and bladder function, nutrition, pain, skin integrity, etc. The MDS helps to identify problem areas for which the treatment team can develop a plan of care. You can view this form and instructions for how to complete it at the CMS website at (www.cms.hhs.gov/CMSForms). For ease and efficiency, each discipline may be assigned a specific part of the MDS to complete. Facilities may vary in how ADL, cognitive, or other sections are divided between occupational therapy, nursing, or other disciplines. Clients are then divided into Resource Utilization Groupings (RUGs) according to how much care they need. This determines the reimbursement that the facility will receive based on the category or level of skilled services required. To substantiate this level of care, each rehabilitation professional might need to document the exact number of therapy minutes provided for each individual client. If this entire process is not done properly, the client will be unable to get the level of care needed. Also, inaccurate assessments and predictions about rehabilitation potential may result in the facility not being reimbursed for care that is provided beyond what was indicated on the MDS.

Specific formats and timelines for occupational therapy documentation will depend on the requirements of the particular facility, accrediting agency, and payment source (Medicare, Medicaid, HMO, etc.). Generally, clients referred to occupational therapy will go through the occupational therapy evaluation process as described in Chapter 12. Subsequent intervention sessions will usually be documented as progress notes at regular intervals, although some facilities may require attendance logs, checklists, or contact notes for each visit. Reevaluation and transition reports are written if needed and according to facility guidelines. An occupational therapy discharge or discontinuation note is written when the client leaves the facility or occupational therapy is no longer necessary.

Outpatient Documentation

Documentation in outpatient settings will also depend on the requirements of the particular facility, accrediting agency, and payment source. Clients referred to outpatient occupational therapy will normally go through the occupational therapy evaluation process as described in Chapter 12. If managed care is involved, the insurance company often provides a special form that the OT fills out outlining the client's problems, reason that skilled occupational therapy is needed, and the plan of care. This is usually in addition to the facility's occupational therapy initial evaluation form. The insurance company may only initially approve a set number of visits within a specified time frame. If additional therapy is needed after those approved visits are completed, a formal request must be made by the therapist. This may involve sending the payment source a progress note or reevaluation report; often this involves another insurance company form that must be completed. Sometimes a phone conversation with the case manager is also needed. Remember to follow HIPAA and facility guidelines at all times in these situations. In outpatient settings, it is especially important to document measurable, objective progress and indicate the limiting factors requiring continued occupational therapy. Your documentation and feedback as an OTA will provide important information to the OT for this purpose.

Depending on the facility, outpatient intervention sessions will usually be documented as progress notes at regular intervals, although some facilities may require attendance logs, checklists, or contact notes for each visit. Reevaluation and transition reports are written as needed and according to facility guidelines and payment source. An occupational therapy discharge or discontinuation note is written when the client leaves the facility or occupational therapy is no longer necessary.

Outpatient Medicare Documentation

Medicare requires that clients receiving outpatient occupational therapy have a certified plan of care (treatment plan). The OT will establish the intervention plan following initial evaluation. This intervention plan is then sent to the referring physician, who reviews it and signs it, indicating approval of the plan. The plan of care at a minimum must include the client's diagnoses, the frequency, duration, type, and amount of OT services, and the occupational therapy long-term goals (CMS, 2005c). Certification means that the client must be under the care of a physician (or approved nonphysician practitioner [NPP]) who must sign this plan of care to certify it for the first 30 days. The plan must then be recertified every 30 days, meaning an updated or modified occupational therapy plan is then reviewed and resigned by the physician/NPP (CMS, 2005d). If a client is receiving multiple rehabilitation services, each discipline must fill out a separate plan of care or Medicare form. As you learned in Chapters 1 and 8, Medicare has strict requirements for what is considered skilled occupational therapy and what is considered necessary and reasonable for the client's condition.

The OT may record the initial assessment for a Medicare client on a Medicare 700 form, which contains spaces to record the client and facility identifying information, medical history, complications that will impact treatment, the reason for referral, and the level of function at the start of care. Medicare no longer requires the use of the 700 form, as long as all the same information is present on the form that the facility chooses to use (CMS, 2003). Progress notes (required every 30 days) may be completed by the OT on a Medicare 701 form, which provides equally small spaces for the reason(s) for continuing treatment for an additional billing period. Documentation should indicate the client's progress, support the reason for continuing skilled occupational therapy, and clarify the occupational therapy goals. The requirement for using the 701 form is also discontinued, as long as all the information on the 701 is present on the form the facility chooses to use (CMS, 2003). The OTA will provide important feedback to the OT for the completion of these forms and may be involved in the mechanics of sending or tracking the paperwork.

As you can see in the examples that follow (Figures 14-1 and 14-2), there is very limited space available for recording data. The examples show the information recorded in the amount of space that is available. In

DEPARTMENT OF HEALTH AND HUMAN SERVICES
CENTERS FOR MEDICARE & MEDICAID SERVICES

PLAN OF TREATMENT FOR OUTPATIENT REHABILITATION
(COMPLETE FOR INITIAL CLAIMS ONLY)

1. PATIENT'S LAST NAME C.	FIRST NAME Rose	M.I. S.	2. PROVIDER NO. XXXXX	3. HICN XXXXX

4. PROVIDER NAME XYZ Care Center	5. MEDICAL RECORD NO. *(Optional)* (Optional)	6. ONSET DATE 4/16/06	7. SOC. DATE 5/05/06

8. TYPE ☐PT ☒OT ☐SLP ☐CR ☐RT ☐PS ☐SN ☐SW	9. PRIMARY DIAGNOSIS *(Pertinent Medical D.X.)* pneumonia, Parkinson's disease	10.TREATMENT DIAGNOSIS 780.9	11. VISITS FROM SOC. 10

12. PLAN OF TREATMENT FUNCTIONAL GOALS

  GOALS *(Short Term)* 2 wks: Client will be: 1. Min Ⓐ in bed mobility with adaptations to use bedside commode. 2. SBA c̄ sit ↔ stand transfers to bed and toilet. 3. Able to ambulate using walker with SBA for safety ↔ bathroom. 4. Propel self in w/c Ⓘ from bedroom to kitchen.
3 wks: Client will be: 1. Min Ⓐ in dressing. 2. Min Ⓐ in bathing.
  OUTCOME *(Long Term)*
6 wks: In order to perform ADL at home, client will be: 1. Ⓘ in mobility & transfers for ADL/IADL. 2. Ⓘ in toileting using bedside commode or bathroom. 3. Ⓘ in w/c mobility. 4. Ⓘ in dressing and bathing.

PLAN
ADL retraining

Transfer training

Functional Mobility training

Safety education

Client/Family education

13. SIGNATURE *(professional establishing POC including prof. designation)* Sally M. OTR/L	14. FREQ/DURATION *(e.g., 3/Wk. x 4 Wk.)* 3/Wk x 6 Wk

I CERTIFY THE NEED FOR THESE SERVICES FURNISHED UNDER THIS PLAN OF TREATMENT AND WHILE UNDER MY CARE ☐ N/A

15. PHYSICIAN SIGNATURE   16. DATE

17. CERTIFICATION
FROM 5/5/06   THROUGH 5/31/06   N/A

18. ON FILE *(Print/type physician's name)*
☐ Dr. Harry H.

20. INITIAL ASSESSMENT *(History, medical complications, level of function at start of care. Reason for referral.)*

19. PRIOR HOSPITALIZATION
FROM 4/16/06   TO 4/19/06   N/A

Client is 73 y.o. f who lived alone and did accounting work until hospitalized for pneumonia 4/16/06. She is now temporarily residing at her daughter's home where she received 2 wks. of home care, including OT. Client was referred to out-pt OT by Dr. H. on 5/3/06 2° to client feeling better. Client states she wants to return home and be Ⓘ in transfers and mobility as in the past. Medical Hx. and complications include Parkinson's disease and several falls. Prior to her illness, client was Ⓘ in bed mobility, ADL, meal & tax preparations. Cognition: alert and oriented x3. ADL tasks: Client mod Ⓐ in bathing and dressing due to fatigue from illness and complications of inactivity and Parkinson's Disease. Client feeds self after set up. Mobility: Client mod Ⓐ in bed mobility supine to sit; min Ⓐ in transfers and requires SBA assistance to ambulate using wheeled walker for safety. She is propelled in w/c by her daughter due to fatigue, balance and ambulation difficulties. AROM is WFL but client is slow to initiate movements. Strength is 4/5 in Ⓑ UEs. Grip strength is 10# on Ⓡ, 8# on Ⓛ. Client is motivated and rehab potential is excellent for return to own home with possible homemaker services or Meals-on-Wheels assistance. Client would benefit from skilled OT instruction in safe use of assistive devices, self-care and IADL, transfer techniques, and home evaluation.

21. FUNCTIONAL LEVEL *(End of billing period)* PROGRESS REPORT   ☐ CONTINUE SERVICES **OR**   ☐ DC SERVICES

22. SERVICE DATES
FROM   THROUGH

Form CMS-700-(11-91)

Figure 14-1. Department of Health and Human Services Form CMS-700.

DEPARTMENT OF HEALTH AND HUMAN SERVICES
CENTERS FOR MEDICARE & MEDICAID SERVICES

UPDATED PLAN OF PROGRESS FOR OUTPATIENT REHABILITATION

(Complete for Interim to Discharge Claims. Photocopy of CMS-700 or 701 is required.)

1. PATIENT'S LAST NAME C.	FIRST NAME Rose	M.I. S.	2. PROVIDER NO. XXXXX	3. HICN XXXXX

4. PROVIDER NAME XYZ Care Center	5. MEDICAL RECORD NO. *(Optional)* *(Optional)*	6. ONSET DATE 4/16/06	7. SOC. DATE 5/05/06

8. TYPE ☐ PT ☒ OT ☐ SLP ☐ CR ☐ RT ☐ PS ☐ SN ☐ SW	9. PRIMARY DIAGNOSIS *(Pertinent Medical D.X.)* pneumonia, Parkinson's disease 12. FREQ/DURATION *(e.g., 3/Wk. x 4 Wk.)* 3/Wk x 4 Wk	10. TREATMENT DIAGNOSIS 780.9	11. VISITS FROM SOC. 10

13. CURRENT PLAN UPDATE, FUNCTIONAL GOALS *(Specify changes to goals and plan.)*

GOALS *(Short Term)*

2 wks: Client will: 1. Ⓘ sit ↔ stand transfers ↔ bed, toilet, and bed-side commode. 2. Manage clothing during dressing, bathing and toileting CGA for balance after set-up. 3. Demonstrate safe transfers and mobility with SBA from daughter during home evaluation. 3 wks: Client will: perform simple stovetop cooking task c̄ SBA and use of walker.

OUTCOME *(Long Term)*

4 wks: In order to perform ADL in her own home, client will be: 1. Ⓘ in bed mobility & transfers. 2. Ⓘ in toileting, dressing and bathing. 3. Ⓘ and safe in use of walker and w/c in home for ADL and light IADL.

PLAN

ADL retraining

Functional mobility

Safety education

Home evaluation

Client/caregiver education

I HAVE REVIEWED THIS PLAN OF TREATMENT AND RECERTIFY A CONTINUING NEED FOR SERVICES. ☐ N/A ☐ DC	14. RECERTIFICATION FROM 6/1/06 THROUGH 6/30/06 N/A
15. PHYSICIAN'S SIGNATURE	16. DATE	17. ON FILE *(Print/type physician's name)* ☐ Dr. Harry H.

18. REASON(S) FOR CONTINUING TREATMENT THIS BILLING PERIOD *(Clarify goals and necessity for continued skilled care.)*

Client has made significant progress in 2 wks. as demonstrated in her ability to sit up in bed and to sit on the side of the bed with CGA using a trapeze bar, a firmer mattress and a small bed rail. Client needs SBA c̄ sit ↔ stand transfers ↔ bed; ambulates using walker c̄ SBA for safety ↔ bathroom. Client now able to propel self in W/C Ⓘ from bedroom to kitchen and bathroom but requires daughter's assistance to go propel w/c outdoors. Demonstrates good awareness of safety precautions by using brakes during transfers. Client progressed from mod to min Ⓐ in dressing and bathing but requires help managing clothing, doing fasteners, and bathing back when standing due to ↓ balance and AROM. Client would benefit from continued ADL retraining, transfer and mobility training using assistive devices, skilled instruction and a home evaluation of mobility and safety issues at home with caregiver assistance. Rehab potential is excellent for discharge to her own apartment in 4-6 wks.

19. SIGNATURE *(or name of professional, including prof. designation)* Sally M., OTR/L	20. DATE 5/31/06	21. ☐ CONTINUE SERVICES **OR** ☐ DC SERVICES

22. FUNCTIONAL LEVEL *(At end of billing period — Relate your documentation to functional outcomes and list problems still present.)*

	22. SERVICE DATES FROM THROUGH

Form CMS-701(11-91)

Figure 14-2. Department of Health and Human Services Form CMS-701.

order for the therapist to include more comprehensive evaluation information, OTs in some facilities fill out the required certification and client identification information on the Medicare forms and attach their own completed regular evaluation and reevaluation forms to it. Other facilities have developed a combined facility/Medicare form to use. This avoids the double paperwork created by completing an evaluation or reevaluation form in addition to a separate Medicare form. As an OTA, it is critical that you understand and adhere to the Medicare guidelines. If the process is not done correctly, your OT services may not be reimbursed.

Acute Care

Occupational therapy practitioners working in acute care settings play a vital role but also face some challenges. These challenges include short lengths of stay, medically fragile clients, and increased productivity demands due to cost saving measures. Discharge planning begins the day the client is admitted and the treatment team provides intervention directed toward the client's needs for the expected discharge environment.

When an order for occupational therapy is received, the evaluation process begins. Occupational therapy may be automatically included as part of clinical pathways for certain diagnoses such as a total hip replacement (McKelvey, 2004). In this case, there are preplanned interventions and goals for each day of the client's hospital stay that can be modified for individual needs. Priorities in occupational therapy should reflect the client's occupational profile. Occupational therapy in acute care normally focuses on basic ADL and activity tolerance (personal hygiene, grooming, self-feeding, transfers), and can also include interventions such as adaptive equipment, energy conservation, and client/caregiver education (McKelvey, 2004). Clients who have orthopedic, neurological, cardiopulmonary or other conditions might also require interventions such as therapeutic exercise programs, positioning, edema management, or splinting, all directed toward the goal of occupational engagement.

Due to the client's rapidly changing status in the acute care environment, contact notes are normally written after each occupational therapy visit. This will communicate important information to the treatment team about any changes in the client's condition, safety, activity tolerance, functional abilities, and barriers to occupational performance. Because of short lengths of stay, formal reevaluation reports are often not necessary. If the client is transferred to another service delivery setting within the organization, a transition plan is written. Otherwise, a discharge or discontinuation note is written when the client is discharged from the facility or occupational therapy is no longer needed.

Home Care

Occupational therapy practitioners in home care work with people of all ages who are considered homebound; that is, the client would have severe difficulty receiving services outside the home. Many of these individuals are elderly clients who have Medicare, so that is what we will discuss in this section. The OT will evaluate the client and establish the intervention plan which delineates what skilled OT services are necessary. The intervention plan will be directed toward the safe and functional daily living skills the client requires in the home environment. OT interventions in home care improve specific BADL, IADL, activity tolerance, safe functional mobility and transfers, and help prevent secondary medical complications. In addition, occupational therapy interventions may include family/caregiver education and recommendations for adaptive equipment or home modifications. Contact notes are written for each visit. In some states, in order for an agency to be certified, the therapist must also provide a written and dated home program in the client's home, with a copy placed in the health record (Shadley and Rexrode, 2005).

The CMS has facilitated the home care industry (including specific disciplines such as occupational therapy) to focus on quality improvement methods for functional client outcomes (Shadley and Rexrode, 2005). One method of gathering outcomes data is through the use of The Outcome and Assessment Information Set (OASIS), which has been required by CMS since 1999 (Shadley and Rexrode, 2005). This client assessment is completed at the start of care, discharge, and at certain other intervals. The OASIS considers the holistic needs of the client such as living situation (safety, hazards), supports, medical status/systems review, ADL, nutrition, mobility, physical functioning, sleep patterns, etc. Each section has a numerical scale and the OASIS may be completed by the RN or rehab therapist (OT, PT, SLP). You can view the OASIS and instructions for how to complete it at the CMS website (www.cms.hhs.gov/CMSForms).

Palliative Care

OTAs who work in hospice or other practice settings where clients have terminal illnesses often provide palliative care rather than rehabilitation. Palliative care involves a philosophy of focusing on providing comfort, symptom relief, emotional support, and quality of life as clients prepare for death. Third party payers look at therapy services slightly differently in these situations. As there is no expectation that the client will make progress in physical functioning, goals often center around quality of life issues such as pain control and maintaining ability to engage in meaningful occupations. Goals might include traditional intervention approaches such as energy conservation, adaptive equipment, positioning, and family/caregiver education. Sometimes nontraditional interventions are also used such as relaxation, active listening, and complementary and alternative therapies.

Different Formats for Notes

Facilities often use checklists, flow sheets, and other similar forms created by the facility instead of SOAP notes to save time. With these other formats, information might be categorized slightly differently than if you are writing a SOAP note. Forms are often a popular way to record an initial assessment because they allow quite a lot of information to be communicated with minimal time spent writing. Narrative notes are not formally organized into sections like SOAP notes. Narrative notes may present any information in any order desired. However, good narrative notes will contain the same type of content in the same basic order, they just will not be delineated as separate SOAP categories and will instead consist of a paragraph format.

Some facilities use DAP notes (Data, Assessment, Plan), which are an adaptation of the SOAP format. In DAP notes, the "D" (data) section contains both the "S" and the "O" information. Other formats of notes include BIRP, PIRP, or SIRP notes. These types of notes are sometimes used in mental health practice settings with the information distributed as follows:

B: The behavior that is exhibited by the client
I: The treatment intervention provided by the OT or OTA
R: The client's response to the intervention provided
P: The therapist's plan for continued intervention, based on the client's response

P: The problem/purpose of the treatment
IRP for intervention, response and plan, as above

S: The situation
IRP for intervention, response, and plan, as above

Electronic Documentation

As productivity standards become more stringent and the healthcare professional's time becomes tighter, the use of electronic technology is rapidly becoming more prevalent. Many facilities are switching to paperless systems and this changes how occupational therapy practitioners approach the documentation process, use specific formats, and communicate with others. As noted in Chapter 2, information can be entered and obtained from different locations and means such as use of handheld devices and the internet. There are many products and software packages available for use in occupational therapy practice that can make our jobs easier, save time, standardize and organize our documentation, and be more cost effective. Some of those may include touch screen or keyboard entry programs for evaluations, clinical notes, conference notes, and plans of care (Nunes, February 22, 2006, personal communication). However, ease of recording and quick access to documents must be weighed against important issues such as security and privacy issues, potential for computer downtime, errors, or accidental destruction of information (Iyer, 2002).

Occupational therapy practitioners might use electronic technology for various functions such as:
- Organizing and managing a schedule
- Communicating with other disciplines, clients, or third party payers
- Sending and receiving documents

- Receiving or requesting orders for occupational therapy
- Reviewing health records
- Recording data and assessment results
- Billing and reimbursement
- Documenting all stages of the intervention process
- Selecting from a standard word bank or menu of problems, goals, and possible intervention strategies specific to a particular practice setting

Occupational therapy practitioners must be careful to avoid a cookbook approach when selecting problems, goals, and interventions from a computer program. Some software programs offer more flexibility than others in terms of customizing formats, and allowing for individual details such as mix-and-match programs or providing places for comments (MacLeod, January 23, 2006, personal communication). Occupational therapy practitioners must always use clinical reasoning and a client-centered approach to carefully establish appropriate and individualized plans of care. As in all aspects of the occupational therapy process, the client must remain our prime focus and we must not lose sight of a client's individual needs or compromise quality care by making the client conform to the specifications of a particular software package.

Now that you have learned the basic requirements for writing notes in different practice settings, it is time to integrate and refine your documentation skills. The next chapter will help you to further practice your skills and make your notes even better.

Chapter 15

___ *Making Good Notes Even Better* ___

This chapter will help you review the four sections of the SOAP note and goal writing. Complete the worksheets to practice what you have learned and improve your skills.

Worksheet 15-1
SOAPing Your Note

Indicate which section of the SOAP note you would place each of the following statements.

_____   Client supine → sit in bed Ⓘ.

_____   Client moved kitchen items from counter to cabinet Ⓘ using Ⓛ hand.

_____   Parent reports child's handwriting has significantly improved within the past month.

_____   Problems include decreased coordination, strength, sensation, and proprioception in left hand which create safety risks in home management tasks.

_____   Client reports that his fingers are stiff this morning and that he is having trouble handling small items like buttons.

_____   By the end of next treatment session, client will be Ⓘ donning/doffing splint.

_____   Client's ↑ of 15 minutes in activity tolerance for UE activities permits her to prepare a light meal Ⓘ.

_____   Child seen in OT clinic to promote development of FM skills for BADL.

_____   In order to return to work, client will demonstrate an increase of 10 lbs. grasp in Ⓛ hand by 1/3/07.

_____   Decreased proprioception and motor planning limit client's ability to dress upper body.

_____   Continue retrograde massage to Ⓡ hand for edema control.

_____   Client's correct identification of inappropriate positioning 100% of the time would indicate memory WFL.

_____   Consumer will be seen 2x weekly to improve task behaviors in order to obtain a job.

_____   Client reports that she cannot remember her hip precautions.

_____   Client would benefit from further instruction to incorporate total hip precautions into lower body dressing, bathing, and hygiene.

_____   Learning was evident by client's ability to improve with repetition.

_____   Client's request to take rest breaks demonstrates knowledge of her limitations in endurance.

_____   Client required 3 verbal prompts to interact with peers in OT social group.

_____   3+ muscle grade of extension in Ⓡ wrist extensors this week shows good progress toward goals.

_____   Client completed weight shifts of trunk x10 in each of anterior, posterior, left and right lateral directions in preparation for standing to perform home management tasks.

_____   Poor temporal organization interferes with getting to work on time.

Writing the "S"—Subjective

This section includes anything significant the client says regarding treatment. When you are working with a young child, a client who is confused or unable to communicate, you may report on nonverbal communication or state what the primary caregiver says. Sometimes inexperienced OTAs simply list anything important the client had to say about his condition but that is not always appropriate. In Worksheet 15-2, all the information is relevant, but does not form a coherent whole. It is better to condense and organize the information to make the "S" more concise.

Worksheet 15-2

Writing the "S"—Subjective

Try to write a more concise version of the following "S."

Client told OTA she has real bad arthritis in her right shoulder and knee.

Client said, "It hurts to stand on my leg."

Client stated, "It [sliding board] needs to be moved further up on the seat."

When asked if she was ok after the transfer, she said "I'm just tired."

Client stated "I'm through" and requested help to get nearer the bed.

When client transferred to the bed, she said, "This is the hardest part."

Client stated she prefers to approach transfers from the affected side.

S:

Writing the "O"—Objective

Your observations are recorded in this section, either chronologically or in categories. Start with a statement of where the client was seen, for how long, and the purpose for the session. The "O" focuses on the client's response to the intervention provided. Remember to deemphasize the treatment media, and accurately describe assist levels. Try to show your professional skill in the first sentence but keep the focus on the client, not the clinician. Consider this example of a client whose limited mobility is compromising his positioning. Rather than saying *Client seen for positioning*, a better choice of an opening sentence would be:

Pt. seen bedside to select positioning strategies to minimize risk of falling out of w/c.

Client seen in home to educate spouse on positioning to prevent skin breakdown.

Client seen in clinic for assessment of w/c positioning to improve sitting posture for mealtimes.

Complete the following worksheet to practice writing good opening lines in the "O" part of the note.

Worksheet 15-3
Making Opening Lines Better

Rewrite the following opening sentences to show how your skill as an OTA is important in each situation.

1. Old opening sentence: Client practiced laundry tasks for 45 minutes.
   Additional information:
   - Client has total hip precautions that raise safety concerns during functional mobility, especially during performance of household chores.
   - Adaptive equipment is available if needed.

2. Old opening sentence: Consumer seen at workshop for 1 hr. to improve job skills.
   Additional information:
   - Deficits in time management skills, which ↓ his ability to work Ⓘ.
   - Bilateral coordination problems interfere with client completing an essential job function of opening/closing boxes.
   - ↓ tolerance to auditory stimuli contributes to client's high distractibility during task completion.

3. Old opening sentence: Client seen in his hospital room bedside for 30 minutes for feeding.
   Additional Information:
   - Client has Ⓛ neglect.
   - Client's dominant hand is flaccid.
   - Adaptive equipment is available.

4. Old opening sentence: Worked with client in kitchen for 1 hr. to ↑ Ⓘ in cooking.
   Additional Information:
   - Client's problems include decreased tolerance for standing and inattention of affected UE, which raise safety concerns.

Be Specific About Assist Levels

Remember that in addition to reporting the level of assistance needed, you also must be specific about **the part of the task** that required assistance.

Not specific enough:

Resident supine → sit with max Ⓐ, sit → stand mod Ⓐ.

Specific:

Resident supine → sit with max Ⓐ to lift legs over EOB, sit → stand with mod Ⓐ for balance and to maintain toe-touch weight bearing precautions with use of walker.

There is a difference between telling why the assist was needed, for example:

Client needed mod verbal cues to eat lunch due to perceptual deficits.

and the part of the task that required assistance, for example:

Client needed mod verbal cues to locate food on Ⓛ side of meal tray.

Make the "O" Complete and Concise

In the objective section of your note, you record your observations of the intervention session. As you become more proficient, it becomes easier to determine what to include and what to omit in order to be concise. Below is an observation of a treatment session that is very concise. Read the note and determine how to improve it before reading on.

Client was seen in hospital room for further ADL training. Client participated in BADL and transfer activities.

BADL

Client donned robe Ⓘ with set-up.
Client donned/doffed socks Ⓘ with set-up.

MOBILITY

Bed → chair with CGA.
Supine → sit Ⓘ.

This note is *too* concise and omits pertinent information. It lacks an indication that skilled occupational therapy was provided. This note could begin with an opening sentence that shows why your skill as an OTA is needed in this situation. As it stands, it is apparent that someone observed the client dress and transfer and recorded assist levels, but nursing staff or a rehabilitation aide could have done this.

Secondly, the activities documented in this note do not appear to require much time, so the session could be very short. If this is an hour treatment session, was anything else done? Was education or special instruction provided? If the client was slow to do the things recorded above, what caused so few activities to take such a long time? Is there a cognitive or perceptual problem? Is there a problem with coordination, safety, or motor planning? Did the client use adapted techniques or adaptive equipment to be Ⓘ?

Third, as this note indicates the client is independent, there is nothing else in this note to justify that additional occupational therapy is necessary. Unless this is the final treatment session, there needs to be information provided that will justify continued treatment.

Mini-Worksheet 15-4: Writing the "O"—Objective

Now it is your turn to practice. Read the observation below and consider what this note needs to make it better. Instead of rewriting the entire note, just write suggestions to improve the note in the box below:

Toilet transfers: max Ⓐ

Toileting: min Ⓐ with SBA 2° inability to support self with Ⓛ arm and to dress

UE dressing :   min Ⓐ, verbal cues, set-up, Ⓘ in pulling shirt over head

LE dressing :   min Ⓐ pants to hips
max Ⓐ pants to waist
modified Ⓘ don Ⓛ shoe (elastic shoelaces)
mod Ⓘ to don Ⓡ shoe

Ⓡ hand status: Ⓡ fingers: small spasticity (index finger greatest amount)
Thumb: cmc joint painful in abd. & flex.
Ⓡ wrist: flaccid

Suggestions to improve this note:

1.

2.

3.

4.

5.

Writing Effective Assessment Statements

It is sometimes difficult for a student or novice OTA to differentiate an observation from an assessment. An observation is anything you see a client do, while your assessment is how it impacts an **area of occupation**. The assessment is your professional opinion about the meaning of what you have just observed in the intervention session. As you analyze the information you gathered, you will look for evidence of problems, progress (or lack of progress), and rehab potential. Problems may include performance skills, client factors, or psychosocial components. The assessment is not the place to include any new information and it should end with a statement of what the client would benefit from. For example, for a client who has hip precautions and for whom you have observed some problem areas, you might say:

A: Client's inability to remember hip precautions without verbal cues during IADL puts her at risk for reinjury. Supportive daughter and ability to use adaptive equipment properly after instruction indicate a good potential for reaching stated goals. Client would benefit from further skilled instruction in maintaining hip precautions during IADL tasks, sit ↔ stand, and transitional living skills.

You have learned a useful formula to assess the underlying factors that are not within functional limits. While not the only correct way to write assessments, this formula will help you to include all the necessary components in your assessment.

Underlying Limiting factor	Functional Impact	Ability to engage in occupation

There are several steps needed to assess an underlying factor that is not within functional limits:

- First determine what the basic deficit or problem is (such as *poor muscle strength* or *inability to attend to task*).
- Make the problem or deficit the subject of your statement for emphasis.
- Determine whether the area of difficulty you have observed today is an indicator of a broader area of occupation. For example, is the decreased strength you observed causing a problem in grooming also creating problems in other basic ADL tasks? Will the client's depressed mood or poor attention cause difficulty with work tasks? Do the problems you observed today create any safety concerns or affect ability to return home?
- Your assessment statement must relate how the problem areas impact the client's ability to engage in meaningful occupation. After each problem you note (e.g., limited strength, poor attention, depressed mood), ask yourself "So what?" So the client is unable to do that—how does this impact his life? The answer to your "So what" question becomes your assessment of the situation.

Let us now compare some observation and assessment statements. Suppose you are working with a client who plans to return home to live alone in her apartment. Your intervention has included teaching her hip precautions following her THR, but she forgets to incorporate these when practicing home management tasks. What is this client's basic or core problem? Why does it matter or why is it important?

The following statement is an objective **observation** of the client's behavior:

Pt was unable to adhere to hip precautions during laundry task due to memory deficit.

However, when phrased differently, it demonstrates the OTA's clinical reasoning and becomes an **assessment** of what was observed:

Memory deficit interferes with client's ability to adhere to total hip precautions, which limits her ability to safely perform self-care and IADL tasks needed to return to prior Ⓘ living situation.

The OTA has determined in the assessment that this client's basic problem is the inability to retain instructions. The OTA should then address this problem with a recommendation to use compensatory techniques (memory cues) of some kind. The safety concerns that impact the client's ability to return home should be considered. Otherwise, why should a third party payer continue to pay for instruction that will not be remembered? According to the formula, rather than repeat what was observed, the assessment begins with the underlying problem, expands the scope of the area of occupation to include related tasks, (in this case IADL and self-care tasks), and answers the question, "So what? Why does this matter in this client's life or why is it important?"

Now compare another observation and assessment:

Observation: *Client's temporal organization was WFL with verbal prompts.*

Assessment: *Client's need for multiple verbal prompts to complete BADL within acceptable time frame indicates probable difficulty for work tasks. Ability to manage time with verbal prompting indicates good potential to reach stated goals.*

Note that in the observation statement, there was no area of occupation mentioned, only a description of task performance. In the assessment statement, you are addressing the area of occupation (work) that is impacted by the underlying factor or problem (decreased temporal organization).

Worksheet 15-5
Differentiating Between Observations and Assessments

Identify which of the statements below are observations, and which are assessments.

_____ Client is unable to don Ⓛ LE prosthesis for functional mobility.

_____ Inability to don Ⓛ LE prosthesis Ⓘ prevents client from performing safe functional mobility around the house to live alone.

_____ Decreased tolerance to auditory stimuli limits the student's ability to attend to classroom tasks.

_____ Student requires verbal cues to stay on task due to decreased tolerance to auditory stimuli.

_____ Client was unable to incorporate relaxation and stress reduction techniques, requiring several verbal prompts to complete task.

_____ Inability to incorporate relaxation and stress reduction techniques when interacting with sales clerk limits her ability to Ⓘ manage shopping tasks p̄ discharge.

Reword the following observations to make them *assessments*.

1. Client demonstrated difficulty with balancing checkbook due to memory and sequencing deficits.

2. Client unable to complete homemaking tasks or basic self-care activities independently due to Ⓛ neglect, impulsive behavior, and decreased attention to task.

3. After use of behavior modification techniques, child demonstrated ability to remain seated at desk for the remainder of the treatment session.

Sweeping Assessment Statements

Due to a busy schedule and time constraints, it can be tempting for an OTA to make brief and sweeping assessment statements such as:

A: Deficits in upper body strength, fine motor, and feeding limit Jordan's ability to be ① in home and classroom activities.

Although accurate, this statement is limited, and would benefit from some elaboration. A better way to assess Jordan's information would be to say:

A: Deficits in upper body strength limit Jordan's ability to be ① in eating, functional mobility, or dressing. Decreased fine motor skills will impede typical classroom activities such as holding a pencil or crayon or manipulating small items, as well as age-appropriate IADL tasks in which Jordan is beginning to show an emerging interest. Jordan would benefit from continued upper body strengthening, reach-grasp-release, and feeding activities to move Jordan more expediently through typical developmental milestones.

The assessment demonstrates your clinical reasoning as an OTA. When you are first learning to write notes, it is helpful to go step by step through your observation data and note the problems, progress, and rehab potential that you see. For any underlying factors not within functional limits, note the areas of occupation these factors are likely to impact.

Worksheet 15-6

Problems, Progress, and Rehab Potential

For the following observation, note the problems or underlying factors not within functional limits. Then list the information that indicates potential for progress.

> *O: Client seen for 30 min. in OT clinic to work on functional movements of Ⓡ UE, dynamic sitting balance, and cognitive skills. Client needed mod Ⓐ in shifting weight to get to edge of w/c and max verbal cues to use correct posture and shift feet during standing pivot transfer w/c → mat. Client requires max verbal cues to initiate grasp of bag in beanbag activity. Client needs mod Ⓐ in reaching with Ⓡ UE. Client demonstrated ability to complete Ⓡ UE shoulder flexion required to toss bag appropriately 2 feet with max verbal cues. Client demonstrated cognitive understanding of activity with mod verbal cues by stating desired goal to be achieved by accurate aim.*

Problems:

Progress/Rehab Potential:

Assessment: How do the problems and progress you noted impact the client's ability to engage in meaningful occupation (such as safety concerns or ability to care for self)? What would the client benefit from? What skilled OT intervention is indicated? Integrate this information to write the "A" part of this note.

A:

Plan: Your plan contains a statement of how often and for how long you will be seeing the client, your priorities and goals. For example:

> *P: Continue tx. 3x wk for 1 wk to work on incorporating hip precautions into ADL tasks. Within 1 week, client will be Ⓘ in IADL tasks following hip precautions 3/3 trials.*

Now finish the note with the plan.

P:

Worksheet 15-7
The "Almost" Note

Now it is your turn to integrate all you have learned. This note is almost good enough. In fact, it appears to be quite good on the surface, but actually has major flaws in organization and clinical reasoning. Mrs. M. is a 78-year-old female who sustained a Ⓛ CVA and has Ⓡ hemiparesis. Her OTA wrote the treatment note below. How can this note be improved? There is no need to try to rewrite the entire note. For this worksheet, simply make suggestions about what this note needs to be more effective.

S: Client reports stiffness in Ⓡ hip, but improvement from previous pain. She states a preference for transferring to her left. Client states that she is willing to do "whatever it takes to get out of the hospital."

O: Client seen in room for work on dressing and functional mobility.

Transfer: Client SBA for standing pivot transfer bed → w/c to the left.
Client min Ⓐ with transfers w/c → toilet using grab bar.

Mobility: Client SBA with VC's to flex trunk when rolling from supine to Ⓡ side.
Client SBA supine → sit; min Ⓐ sit → stand.
Client Ⓘ in w/c mobility.

Dressing: Client Ⓘ in donning shirt.
Client min Ⓐ with VC's to don bra while standing.
Client Ⓘ in donning socks and shoes.
Client min Ⓐ with walker and VC in donning underwear and pants.
Client needs setup for dressing activities.

UE ROM: Ⓛ UE – WFL.
Ⓡ UE – ↓ range in proximal shoulder flexion.

Static standing: Client CGA with walker Ⓑ UE support.

Dynamic standing: Client SBA with walker for balance.

A: Deficits noted in Ⓡ UE coordination, Ⓑ UE strength, and dynamic standing balance. Client Ⓘ in dressing EOB, but is min Ⓐ in dressing when standing with a walker. Ⓛ UE AROM is WFL but Ⓡ UE has deficits noted in shoulder flexion. Client needs SBA in bed mobility when rolling to unaffected side and min Ⓐ in sit → stand 2° ↓ UE strength. Client needs SBA for transfer to unaffected side in pivot transfer bed → w/c and min Ⓐ w/c → toilet. Client would benefit from skilled OT to continue UE strengthening and coordination exercises and to ↑ dynamic standing balance using walker, in order to ↑ Ⓘ in ADL.

P: Client to be seen twice daily for 30-minute sessions to continue to work on dynamic standing balance. Client will require SBA in grooming activities standing sink-side with standard walker within 2 weeks.

List suggestions for improving the Almost Note:

Worksheet 15-8
Writing Functional and Measurable Goals

The FEAST method is useful to make sure that you include all the necessary components when writing goals and objectives.

F: Function (If not embedded in the action)	For what functional gain?
E: Expectation	The client will..?
A: Action	Do what?
S: Specific Conditions	Under what conditions?
T: Timeline	By when?

However, writing the components in that order sometimes leads to a very awkward sentence. Try rewriting the following goals in a more logical order, making sure that the FEAST components are present in the goal statement.

Client will pivot while standing with SBA during toilet transfers in 1 day.

Client will be min Ⓐ in dressing UE and LE in 10 days.

It is important to de-emphasize the treatment media when writing your goals. Rewrite the following goal statements to emphasize the changes in performance skills you would like to see while de-emphasizing the treatment interventions you are using.

Client will place 8 half-inch screws and washers on a block of wood with holes by next treatment session.

Client will make a clock using the appropriate materials while sitting by anticipated discharge in 1 week.

Client will stay in his chair without reminders and spend at least 30 minutes lacing the leather billfold during the 45-minute craft group session in 2 weeks.

Conclusion

Congratulations! If you have read all the material presented in this manual and completed all the exercises, you should be able to document your client care according to the most rigorous standards. You are well on your way to becoming an OTA. The following notes are intended to provide you with examples of well-written notes from a variety of practice settings. These examples, along with the ones imbedded in the various chapters, should provide you with ideas for documenting some of the more common kinds of treatment sessions. Remember that occupational therapy practitioners have different writing styles and that there is more than one "correct" way to state the same information. If you work in a setting that is not represented, you are invited to contribute notes to the next edition of this manual.

We welcome your comments, criticisms, ideas, and suggestions for ways to make this book better or more useful to instructors, students, and beginning OTAs. We also invite you to submit examples of documentation that you consider to be good examples of some particular concept (such as conciseness). We are particularly interested in notes that represent best practice in occupational therapy today.

When submitting a note, please include your name, address, and telephone number, along with your permission to publish the note. Please send your comments, suggestions, or notes to:

Sherry Borcherding, OTR and Marie J. Morreale, OTR
c/o SLACK Incorporated
Health Care Books and Journals
6900 Grove Road
Thorofare, NJ 08086

The insert at the back of the book summarizes everything you have learned about writing occupational therapy SOAP notes. Pull it out and carry it with you to use as a quick and easy reference guide while you are learning and practicing your professional documentation skills.

A Quick Checklist for Evaluating Your Note

Use the following summary chart as a quick reference guide to be sure that your note contains all the essential elements.

S: Subjective

☐ 1. Use something significant the client says about his treatment or condition

O: Objective

☐ 1. Begin this section with length of time, where and for what the client was seen.

☐ 2. Report what you see, either chronologically or using categories,

☐ 3. Remember to do the following:
- Deemphasize the media
- Specify what the part of the task the assistance was for
- Show skilled OT happening
- Leave yourself out
- Focus on the client's response
- Avoid being judgmental

A: Assessment

☐ 1. Look at the data in your "O" sentence by sentence, asking yourself what problems, progress, and rehab potential you see.

☐ 2. Ask yourself "So what?" Why is this important in the client's life? For each underlying factor not within functional limits, identify the impact it will have on an area of occupation

☐ 3. End the "A" with "client would benefit from..."
- Justify continued skilled OT
- Set up the plan

(Be sure the time lines and activities you are putting in your plan match the skilled OT you say your client needs.)

P: Plan

☐ 1. Specify how often the client will be seen and for how long.

☐ 2. Tell what you will be working on during that time

☐ 3. End with a LTG or STG, whichever is more appropriate for your client & practice setting

☐   Make certain engagement in occupation is integral to the note.

☐   Make certain everything goes together. For example, if you talk about inability to dress in the problem list, don't switch to feeding in the goals and showering in the plan.

☐   Remember to sign and date your note.

If you have read the text carefully you will understand what each item means. For a more complete explanation, refer to the chapter that provides information in detail. There is a brief explanation of SOAP guidelines on the back of this sheet.

"S" Subjective

☐   Use something significant the client says about his treatment or condition.

☐   If there is nothing significant, ask yourself whether you are using your interview skills to elicit the information about how the client sees things.

"O" Objective

☐   Begin this section with length of time, where the client was seen and for what reason. For example:

Client seen for 30 minutes bedside for functional mobility

☐   Report what you see, either chronologically or using categories.

☐   Remember to do the following:

  ☐ Focus on performance elements & deemphasize the media. For example:

  Client worked on tripod pinch using pegs.

  ☐ When giving assist levels, specify the part of the task the assistance was for.

  Client min Ⓐ for correct hand placement during pivot transfer to toilet.

  ☐ Show skilled OT happening—make it clear that you were not just a passive observer.

   For example, don't just list all the assist levels and think that is enough.

  ☐ Write from the client's point of view, leaving yourself out.

  Client repositioned rather than *OTA repositioned the client.*

  ☐ Focus on the client's response, rather than on what you did.

  Client able to don socks using dressing stick after demonstration.

  ☐ Avoid being judgmental.

  For example, say client *"...didn't complete the activity."* Don't add " *...because he was stubborn."*

"A" Assessment

☐   Look at the data in your "O" sentence by sentence, identifying problems, progress, and rehab potential. Ask yourself what each statement means for the client's occupational performance. This is your assessment of the data. For example, if in your "O" you noted that client falls to the left when sitting unsupported, what do you think this means he will be unable to do for himself? For example: *Client unable to sit EOB unsupported to dress.*

☐   Be sure you have not introduced any new information.

☐   End the "A" with "client would benefit from..."

☐   Justify continued skilled OT: *Client would benefit from skilled instruction in energy conservation techniques as well as continued work on AROM of the UEs, strengthening, and compensatory techniques for performing IADL tasks one handed.*

☐   Set-up the plan. (Be sure the time lines you are putting in your plan match the skilled OT you document that your client needs.) For example, if you justify skilled OT by saying only, *Client would benefit from skilled instruction in energy conservation techniques*, then do not say that you plan to treat him twice a day for 2 weeks. Skilled instruction in energy conservation should take only one session, or at most two sessions.

"P" Plan

☐   Specify frequency and duration of treatment: *Continue tx. one hour daily for 2 weeks.*

☐   Identify the specific performance areas that will be addressed during that time: *Client to continue OT one hour daily for 2 weeks for instruction in Ⓘ in bathing, grooming, and hygiene.*

☐   End with a LTG or STG, whichever is more appropriate for your client and the practice setting: *By the end of the week, client will be able to don socks Ⓘ sitting EOB without losing balance.*

Chapter 16

Examples of Different Kinds of Notes

This final chapter provides examples of notes from different stages of treatment and from a variety of practice settings. The first group of notes illustrates different stages of the intervention process, while the second set provides examples of single treatment sessions in different practice settings.

Examples of Notes for Different Stages of Treatment

Acute Care Hospital: Initial Evaluation Report (including intervention plan)
Outpatient Rehabilitation: Cancer Intervention Plan
Progress Note: Hand Therapy Clinic
Progress Note: Inpatient Mental Health
Acute Care Hospital Discharge Note: (SOAP Format)
Discharge Note: (Facility Format)

Examples of Treatment Notes for Different Kinds of Treatment Sessions

Contact Note: Acute Care
Contact Note: Safety
Contact Note: Cognition
Contact Note: Home Health Visit
Contact Note: Inpatient Mental Health
Contact Note: Pediatric (Preschool Age)
Contact Note: Public School
Contact Note: Outpatient Clinic–Splint
Contact Note: Wheelchair Mobility Instruction

Most of the notes in this section (and in other parts of this manual) were written by students, faculty, and practicing therapists. The signatures, names, and other information have been modified or fabricated to make the notes anonymous. You may assume that demographic data not present on a contact note is stamped by addressograph card onto the page.

Acute Care Hospital: Initial Evaluation Report

Name: Rebecca B.   **Age**: 80   **Primary Dx**: Fx. Ⓛ hip   **Secondary Dx**: Hypertension
Primary payment source: Medicare   **Secondary payment source**: none
Admission date: 9/2/06   **Date of Referral**: 9/3/06
Estimated length of stay: 4 days   **Physician**: B. Garrett, MD
Brief Occupational Profile: Ms. B. reports living alone and being Ⓘ in all ADL prior to admission. She had gone upstairs to use the bathroom because there was none on the first floor. She became lightheaded, fell down the stairs and broke her hip. She was admitted for a total hip replacement yesterday. Her husband died 3 years ago and her family lives out of town and cannot stay with her. She wants to return home. Ms. B has supportive neighbors and lives in a small town where she is retired from her position as second grade teacher. She lives in a townhouse across the street from the elementary school. She is in the habit of visiting with the children and some of their families when school is out each day. She is also active in church activities and belongs to the choir.

Date: 9/3/06   **Time**: 8:30 AM   Occupational Therapy Note

S: Client stated that she would like to "get this leg well" and go home to "live a regular life."

O: Client seen in room for initial evaluation of morning ADL capabilities after Ⓛ THR. Client educated on use of ADL equipment for self-care tasks and adherence to hip precautions. Client demonstrated ability to repeat 2/4 precautions. During ADL evaluation client was observed flexing 8°- 10° beyond 90° and required 4 verbal cues to remain at or below 90° during the 45-minute session. Other 3 hip precautions were followed Ⓘ. Client able to complete sponge bath at sink p̄ set-up for upper body, and used dressing stick with washcloth and verbal cues for lower body. Client PWB on Ⓛ leg; required min Ⓐ for balance with sit ↔ stand to bathe back peri area. Client able to complete upper body dressing after set-up. Client able to don underwear and pants over hips using a dressing stick. Client able to don socks using sock aid after set-up with verbal cues. Client able to complete grooming tasks and oral care Ⓘ. Following verbal cues, client demonstrated good problem solving by trying different body positions to perform ADL while adhering to hip precautions and demonstrated understanding of adaptive aids by utilizing reacher and dressing stick correctly after instruction. Client demonstrated ↓ ADL tolerance as she required four 2-minute rest breaks during dressing tasks. Client then seen in OT clinic for evaluation of client factors:

Ⓑ UE AROM – WFL   Ⓑ UE strength – WFL
UE sensation – intact   Grip strength Ⓡ 47#, Ⓛ 43# (Ⓡ hand dominant)
Tripod pinch Ⓡ 10#, Ⓛ 5#   Lateral pinch Ⓡ 10#; Ⓛ 5#

A: Client demonstrated good motivation, problem solving skills and understanding of equipment use. Upper body strength and AROM WFL, all of which indicate excellent rehab potential. Although she is able to complete grooming tasks and oral care Ⓘ, client is unsafe to complete lower body dressing and bathing due to ↓ endurance, ↓ balance and inconsistent compliance with hip precautions. Problem areas include ↓ balance in sit ↔ stand, ↓ ADL activity tolerance, and ↓ safety in ADL tasks. These problem areas negatively impact client's ability to be Ⓘ and safe in ADL tasks. Client would benefit from skilled instruction on hip precautions and use of adaptive equipment with ADL performance, therapeutic activities which facilitate dynamic standing balance and ↑ ADL activity tolerance. Exploration of interim living arrangement or possible continued home visits and home equipment procurement if progress warrants discharge to home.

P: Client to be seen twice daily for 1 hour the next 3 days to ↑ Ⓘ in self-care tasks through instruction on hip precautions and use of adaptive equipment, with tasks to ↑ activity tolerance, and balance activities using reaching patterns while standing.

LTG: By anticipated discharge on 9/7/06 client will:
1. Safely complete lower body dressing and bathing modified ① utilizing adaptive equipment with 100% adherence to hip precautions.
2. Be ① and safe in toileting using adaptive equipment (walker & bedside commode).

STG: By 4th tx. session client will:
1. Demonstrate ability to don shoes & socks 100% of time ①, utilizing adaptive techniques & devices with 100% adherence to hip precautions.
2. ↑ ADL tolerance as demonstrated by no more than one 15 sec. rest break during lower body dressing task of donning slacks.
3. Safely bathe her peri area modified ① utilizing adaptive techniques and devices with 100% adherence to hip precautions.

By next tx. session client will transfer with SBA sit ↔ stand using bedside commode and manage clothing with no more than 2 verbal cues.

By 2nd tx. session client will be ① in sit ↔ stand using walker.

By 3rd tx. session client will be assessed for possible continued home visits and home equipment procurement if progress warrants discharge to home.

Signature: Kim N., OTR/L

Intervention Plan

Name: Rebecca B.   **Age**: 80   **Primary Dx**: Left hip fracture/THR   **Secondary Dx**: HTN
Strengths: UE strength & AROM WFL; intact cognition and motivation to return home

---

Functional Problems: Unsafe in ADL tasks due to ↓ compliance with hip precautions following THR, ↑ fatigue, ↓ endurance for ADL tasks requiring frequent rest breaks

Long-term Goals	Short-term Goals	Treatment Interventions
By discharge (9/7/06) client will safely complete LE dressing and bathing utilizing adaptive equipment with 100% adherence to hip precautions.	By 9/5/06 client will: 1. Demonstrate ability to don shoes & socks 100% of time with no verbal cues, utilizing adaptive techniques & devices with 100% adherence to hip precautions.	Instruct and have client verbalize 4/4 hip precautions. Instruct in use of adaptive techniques /devices followed by demonstration of use in dressing and bathing activities.
	2. ↑ ADL tolerance as demonstrated by no more than one 15 sec. rest break during dressing task of donning slacks.	Educate client & provide written instructions on energy conservation techniques. Evaluate understanding by her application during ADL tasks; ask about how she performs ADL tasks at home.
	3. Safely bathe her peri area utilizing adaptive techniques and devices with 100% adherence to hip precautions.	Instruct in manipulation of clothing and bathing items while standing in walker at sink s̄ violating hip precautions.

Functional Problem: ↓ dynamic balance makes client unsafe during ADL tasks

By discharge (9/7/06) client will be Ⓘ and safe in toileting using adaptive equipment (walker and bedside commode).	1. Client Ⓘ in sit ↔ stand using walker in 2 tx. sessions while observing total hip precautions.	Instruct client in safe transfer techniques; reinforce compliance with total hip precautions.
	2. Client will transfer with SBA sit ↔ stand using bedside commode and manage clothing with no more than 2 verbal cues by next tx. session.	Provide UE strengthening through reaching and wt. bearing activities at sink and closet for grooming and dressing items and pushing up from chair and bedside commode.
	3. Client will be assessed for possible continued home visits and home equipment procurement if progress warrants discharge to home by 3rd tx. session.	Interview client regarding home environment; explore and discuss interim living arrangements or possible equipment use & placement in home; discuss support services needed if discharge home is warranted.

Discharge Plan: To assisted living facility for 3 to 4 wks. until safe in completing all ADL tasks Ⓘ at home with assistance of home health aide if warranted by progress.

Outpatient Rehabilitation: Cancer Intervention Plan

Name: Carol M.   **Age**: 35   **Primary Dx**: Ⓛ mastectomy 2° breast CA
Strengths: Prior to surgery Carol was in good physical condition and employed full time as a library clerk. She has some social support from her sister who lives in another state.

Functional Problem:
Carol avoids social outings with friends due to ↓ self-esteem secondary to cosmetic alterations imposed by mastectomy procedure, which precludes her ability to return to work.

Long-Term Goal:
Carol will ↑ social interactions and activity to 6 outings/month within the next month, in preparation for return to work.

Objectives	Interventions
STG: Carol will identify one support group of interest to her within 1 week in order to ↑ willingness to be out in public for work and social activities.	Educate Carol re: available support groups and peer visitation groups, their contact persons, telephone numbers, and ask her whether or not she has made contact.
STG: Carol will attend 1 support group activity within 2 weeks in order to ↑ confidence in social and work situations.	Discuss Carol's experiences with the support groups.
STG: Carol will initiate conversation with at least one other support group member during her first visit to the group in order to ↓ negative impact of cosmetic alterations to body image.	Accompany Carol into the community the first time she goes out.
STG: Carol will enroll in a women's exercise program in order to ↑ activity tolerance and positive body image.	Educate Carol re: area exercise groups for post-mastectomy clients.
STG: Carol will identify 5 assets she possesses other than physical in order to ↑ self-esteem and confidence in social and work situations.	Discuss Carol's assets with her, encouraging her to think of as many as she can.

Functional Problem Statement: Carol is unable to return to work 2° 3/4 AROM, 4-/5 muscle strength, ↓ activity tolerance (fatigues after 1 hr.), and sensory changes.

Long-Term Goal: Carol will return to work part-time by 8/8/06.

Objectives	Interventions
STG: Carol will demonstrate activity tolerance of 2 hours for work tasks within 3 weeks.	Scar massage and myofacial release to incision area along with client education on self-massage.
STG: Carol will demonstrate ↑ of 20 ° in Ⓛ shoulder flexion in order to be able to reach the items she needs to work.	PROM to Ⓛ shoulder -- instruct in self ranging program. Active resistive ROM to Ⓛ UE.
STG: Carol will demonstrate strength of 5- in Ⓛ shoulder musculature in order to be able to complete repetitive tasks at work.	Resistive strengthening with thera-tubing, weights, and graded functional activities. Work simulation with client education on energy conservation principles. Provide home exercise program and modify as client progresses. Provide education on women's exercise groups.
STG: Carol will use correct body mechanics in seated and active work tasks in order to have pain level of < 2/10 while working.	Educate in ergonomics and posture in order to prevent pain.
STG: Carol will observe sensory precautions in work and daily living tasks.	Provide education on safety concerns with sensory loss.

Progress Note: Hand Therapy Clinic

Date: 9/11/06   **Time**: 1:00 PM   Occupational Therapy Progress Note

S: Client reports pain @ the ulnar styloid with forearm supination. Client reports she is still unable to start her car c̄ her Ⓡ hand but can now use it to turn a doorknob.

O: Client seen in hand clinic for functional range of motion in Ⓡ UE. Moist heat applied to Ⓡ hand and forearm for 10 minutes prior to beginning treatment.
A/PROM measurements for Ⓡ hand and forearm are:

[KEY: flexion/extension; ( ) PROM; - extension lag; + hyperextension]

Ⓡ hand	MP	PIP	DIP
Index	0/90	0/105	0/75
Long	0/90	0/105	0/80
Ring	0/90	0/105	0/80
Small	0/90	-14/105 (0/105)	0/79

Ⓡ Wrist: +45/40 composite   (+60/50) composite   +45/50 non-composite
Ⓡ forearm: supination 62 (78)   Pronation 90

Client performed the following exercises c̄ Ⓡ UE:
Isometric forearm supination x10, AAROM supination x5, AROM forearm supination x5. After exercise, client's supination ↑ to 77° AROM. HEP revised to include blue foam for flexion strengthening 2 to 3x day.

A: Client's gains in DIP flexion AROM since last week is due to ↑ strength of flexors. Active wrist extension ↑ 9° and extension ↑ 5° from last week. ↑ in active pronation is due to ↑ strength while client lost 14° of forearm supination since last week which appears to be a result of muscle tightness. Client would benefit from continued skilled OT to regain functional AROM to complete IADL and for general strengthening.

P: Client to be seen 2 x wk. for 30 minute sessions. Continue wrist exercises and modify treatment plan to include more supination stretching and strengthening. Client will demonstrate Ⓘ in HEP and sufficient ↑ in Ⓡ forearm supination to start her car c̄ Ⓡ UE in 2 weeks.

Laurie D., COTA

Progress Note: Inpatient Mental Health

Date: 9/21/06   **Time**: 1600   Occupational Therapy Note

S: During the first 2 days of admission, Ms. Jones elected not to attend OT group sessions, maintaining that she was too "anxious and overwhelmed."

O: Client stayed in her room most of the time for first 2 days despite consistent invitations to attend groups. On this day the client attended a stress management group. Initially she was quiet, but gradually began entering into the activity. She was able to identify specific physical, emotional, and behavioral symptoms that she experiences when feeling overwhelmed or anxious. Ms. Jones stated that she had not been aware of these stress reactions.

A: The client is making progress as indicated by her initiating attendance to group, as well as relaxing and opening up socially during the group. Additional progress indicated by recognizing specific symptoms of stress as opposed to relating only general feelings.

P: Continue all goals as originally stated. Client to be seen daily for 1 week to provide opportunities for Ms. Jones to learn basic stress management techniques so that she may recognize and control stress reactions when she begins feeling overwhelmed or anxious.

David L., COTA

Acute Care Hospital: Discharge Note (SOAP Format)

Client: Ted D.   **Admit Date**: 8/29/06   **OT order received**: 9/7/06
OT Evaluation completed: 9/8/06   **Number of treatments**: 5
Discharge Date: 9/16/06

S: Client reports "doing a lot better" and being "less confused" than he was on admission.

O: Client initially presented with multiple trauma 2° to MVA. OT evaluation on 9/8/06 indicated client had deficits in short-term memory, safety awareness, attention to task, and ADL status. Client seen 30 minutes daily for 5 days for ADL retraining for dressing and grooming and functional mobility. Client and family received skilled instruction in safety precautions in the home. Client's functional status on admit and discharge as follows:

Goal # Admit status	Goal	Discharge status
#1 Min Ⓐ in grooming	set up/supervision	set up/supervision
#2 CGA in toilet transfers	SBA	SBA
#3 Supine → sit with min Ⓐ	SBA	SBA
#4 Min Ⓐ UE dressing	set up/supervision	set up/supervision

A: All goals achieved due to improved cognitive status, awareness of safety precautions, and skilled instruction in ADL. Client will need supervision at home 2° remaining cognitive (attention and short-term memory) deficits.

P: Client discharged to home. Recommend home health OT evaluation for safety in home environment and potential for necessary durable medical equipment. No home exercise program given. No other referrals at time of discharge. OT will follow-up in 1 month by phone to check client's functional status in the home.

Laura P., OTR/L

Discharge Note (Facility Format)

Name: Marjorie P.   **Health Record**: # 97865
Physician: Harry H., MD   **Start of Care**: 7/1/06
Room: # 537   **Date of Discharge**: 7/10/06
Primary Dx: Ⓡ CVA   **Secondary Dx**: Arthritis

X Occupational Therapy   _ Physical Therapy   _ Communicative Disorders

Course of treatment: Client seen daily for 9 days, 30 minutes each session following CVA to work on ↑ independence in self-care skills, functional mobility, UE strengthening, energy conservation, & activity tolerance.

Status on Discharge: Client reports feeling much better and is ready to go home.

Discharge Status   Admit status
Self-care Ⓘ and safe   Self-care mod Ⓐ
Functional mobility Ⓘ and safe   Functional mobility mod Ⓐ
Activity tolerance 7 minutes for ADL tasks   Activity tolerance 10 minutes for ADL tasks

Goals met: Client has met self-care and functional mobility goals using energy conservation techniques.

Goals not met: Activity tolerance goal not met due to client declining last 2 treatment sessions when she learned she was being discharged.

Client/Family education: Client instructed in and demonstrates understanding of HEP. Handouts given. Client reports having weights at home she can use for continued UE strengthening as instructed in her HEP.

Recommendations: Discharge client to her sister's home due to goals being met. HEP attached. No home health recommended at this time.

Bonnie B., OTR/L

Contact Note: Acute Care

Date: 8/22/06   **Time**: 15:00   Occupational Therapy Contact Note

S: Client nonverbal. Client demonstrated startle response $\bar{c}$ position change.

O: Client seen bedside to work on initiating and attending to self-care task. When asked to point finger, client required multiple verbal cues and demonstrations, and demonstrated poor response time. Client requires max Ⓐ supine → sit EOB. Client required multiple verbal cues and hand over hand Ⓐ 75% of the time to initiate holding on to wash cloth. Client able to bring wash cloth to water with one verbal cue but required hand over hand Ⓐ to bring wash cloth to face. Client attended to looking at self in mirror for ~ 1 minute. Client required hand over hand Ⓐ to initiate brushing hair. Shoulder AROM limited due to ↑ tone.

A: Overall, client's motor planning, task initiation, and attention during treatment activities continues to be limited. Client would benefit from ranging activities to increase shoulder elevation, as well as further interventions focusing on the skills of initiating and attending to task in order to complete ADL activities.

P: Client to continue OT daily for 20 minute sessions until discharge in ~ 4 weeks to work on self-care activities and the underlying performance skills and client factors necessary to complete tasks Ⓘ. Client will follow a one-step command in 1 week in order to attend to self-care routine.

Susan S., COTA

Contact Note: Safety

Date: 8/29/06   **Time**: 8:45 AM   Occupational Therapy Contact Note

S. Client stated he desires to return home and does not understand why he needs "so much therapy."

O. Client seen bedside for instruction in ADL, use of adaptive equipment, and safety. As client was instructed in method for transfer from bed to w/c, he impulsively attempted to get out of bed before OTA initiated procedure. He required mod Ⓐ to safely sit in w/c 2° poor balance. Meal tray placed on w/c lapboard and client was instructed in use of non skid matting and scoop dish for cereal. Client required mod verbal cues to locate items on Ⓛ side of food tray and to use Ⓛ UE as a functional assist when opening containers and holding breakfast sandwich. Mod verbal cues also were required for pacing of feeding as client pocketed food in Ⓛ cheek and drank liquids too quickly.

A. Client's Ⓛ neglect and poor safety awareness create concerns for returning home. Poor safety awareness while eating poses risk for aspiration and necessitates constant supervision during meals. His improved motor return and ability to use Ⓛ UE as a functional assist with verbal cues will ↑ ability to manage bimanual tasks. Client would benefit from compensatory techniques and activities to ↓ Ⓛ neglect and ↑ safety awareness for ADL.

P. Continue OT twice daily for 45-min sessions to improve safety for transfers, feeding, and self-care. Post written safety reminders bedside, instruct in proper pacing and swallowing of food, and continue to work on sequencing and Ⓛ side awareness. By 9/5/06, client will locate items on food tray with min verbal cues and will verbalize safety reminders for feeding with two verbal cues to look at and read safety list.

Jane D., COTA
Claire T., OTR/L

Contact Note: Cognition

Date: 9/5/06   **Time**: 10:00 AM   Occupational Therapy Note

S: Veteran reports feeling fine, but says he does not remember the OTA's name that he has been working with.

O: Veteran seen in OT clinic for cognitive tasks, Ⓡ UE AROM, strengthening and fine motor coordination. Veteran oriented to person, month, year, and place after prompting. He followed two-step commands after max verbal cues and mod physical assist to complete basic self-care tasks. Veteran was unable to grasp and release items with Ⓡ hand. He required mod physical Ⓐ and verbal cues to complete UE AROM used in table top activities.

A: Veteran is not oriented to surroundings at all times, which presents safety concerns. His ↓ cognitive functioning leads to ↓ attention to completion of tasks, specifically dressing, feeding, and bathing. Veteran would benefit from cognitive skills training and safety instruction. Veteran also displays ↓ strength, coordination, and AROM in Ⓡ UE which limits his ability to complete ADL activities. He would benefit from instruction in using Ⓡ UE as an assist as well as from activities to ↑ Ⓡ UE strength, AROM, and coordination to perform self-care activities.

P: Veteran will be seen daily for 4 weeks for 1 hour to improve cognitive skills, ↑ attention to task and safety awareness, and to ↑ Ⓡ UE strength, AROM, and coordination in order to complete self-care tasks. Veteran will attend to task for 10 minutes in order to complete morning grooming within 2 weeks.

Duane T., COTA
Patty N, OTR/L

Contact Note: Home Health Visit

Home Health Agency
Visit Note

Date: 7/4/06   **Time**: 9:30 AM   Occupational Therapy Note

S: Client stated that he did not sleep well last night and is feeling tired this morning. Client's daughter reported that client is "transferring a little better."

O: Client seen in his home for skilled instruction in ADL, safety, transfers, and use of adaptive equipment. Client and daughter were instructed in use of transfer tub bench. Following demonstration, daughter demonstrated ability to safely transfer client w/c ↔ tub bench with client needing min assist for balance and to bring legs over edge of tub. Following set up, client was able to sequence steps for bathing but required min assist to wash back and feet using long handle sponge. Recommended to client and daughter that grab bar be installed in tub area.

A: Client demonstrates good progress in transfers from mod to min Ⓐ as compared to last week. Client's daughter demonstrates good carryover in safe transfer techniques. Client would benefit from further skilled OT instruction in transfers, self-care activities, and adaptive equipment to increase Ⓘ in home environment.

P: Client to be seen 2x wk. for 45-min sessions to continue work on transfers, self-care Ⓘ, and family education. Client will demonstrate transfers to tub bench Ⓘ with use of grab bar within three treatment sessions.

Jeanine F., COTA
Leah S., OTR/L

Contact Note: Inpatient Mental Health

Date: 4/16/06   **Time**: 4:00 pm   Occupational Therapy Note

S: Client reported she is currently not volunteering and has not worked for the past 4 years due to her disability status. Regarding volunteering, she says "I need the structure," and further stated that she wants to be productive. Currently, client reports she sleeps "too much," and is having relationship problems.

O: Client was admitted yesterday and attended 4/4 group sessions today. During expressive therapy group, client participated in baking with the rest of the group, but did not eat anything. When each group member identified current emotions, client identified hers as miserable, angry, very anxious, overstimulated, frustrated, frightened, and alienated. During skills group, client identified a possible problem she may encounter upon discharge to be lack of organization, with her "red flags" being oversleeping and agitation. Client welcomed suggestions from others restructuring her use of time.

A: Client is very perceptive of her emotions and limitations. Her refusal to eat with the group indicates continued appetite disturbance. Client would benefit from information about eating disorders. She would also benefit from continued group participation, with emphasis on increasing self esteem and time management skills. Client's participation in all 4 group sessions today indicates good rehab potential.

P: Client will continue to attend all daily group sessions while on the acute unit to work on increasing self-esteem and ability to structure her time. Client will demonstrate increased time management skills by naming five strategies she will use for gaining control of her daily time by discharge in approximately 4 days.

Nancy B., OTR/L

Contact Note: Pediatric (Preschool Age)

Date: 4/7/06   **Time**: 3 PM   Occupational Therapy Note

S: Mary said she wanted to play, but when the task was difficult for her, she said, "You do it. You fix it."

O: Mary seen in her home to work on Ⓑ use of UE to ↑ spontaneous use of Ⓛ hand as a functional assist, sitting balance while tailor sitting unsupported, and functional mobility, as a prerequisite to self-care and play skills. Mary was engaged during ~ 90% of the session.
<u>Bilateral UE Use</u>: Mary required max Ⓐ to pull shirt over stuffed animal's arms with Ⓡ UE while holding it with Ⓛ UE. She spontaneously used Ⓛ hand to assist with stabilizing animal while pulling sleeve over its arm and shoulder c̄ Ⓡ hand. Mary initiated snapping shirt, but needed max Ⓐ to use Ⓛ hand to stabilize shirt while fastening snaps. Ⓑ hands used to hold animal steady during play.
<u>Sitting Balance</u>: Mary requires touch cues from stand → sit in walker and mod physical Ⓐ from side sit → cross legged sit. She demonstrated adequate sitting balance to play for 5 minutes, requiring tactile cues twice to right herself from a lateral tilt.

A: Mary demonstrated Ⓑ coordination and use of Ⓛ hand as a functional assist ~ 60% of the time, which is an increase from last week. When she is engrossed in activity, Mary is unable to concentrate on postural support, and needs CGA assist to resume upright posture. She would benefit from continued skilled OT for activities which challenge postural support in order to gain protective responses, body righting, and vestibular integration in order to ↑ her Ⓘ during play.

P: Mary will be seen weekly for 7 weeks to continue strengthening postural support in order to ↑ her Ⓛ in play activities, promote Ⓑ hand use and ↑ use of the Ⓛ hand as a functional assist during ADL and play activities. Mary will be able to maintain upright posture for 10 minutes without lateral tilt within 3 weeks.

Julie S., OTR/L

Contact Note: Public School

Date: 5/12/06 **Time**: 2:30 pm Occupational Therapy Note

S: Heather did not use verbal language to communicate, but did echo words spoken to her.

O: Heather was seen in classroom to work on fine motor skills to prepare for scissors use and improve prehension patterns for writing. After 5 minutes of brushing to decrease tactile sensitivity, Heather worked on palmar pinch and tripod grasp prehension patterns using a "Fruit Loop" bracelet activity for 20 minutes. Heather used tongs (in preparation for scissors use) to pull 15 Fruit Loops out of a cup one at a time. Then using a palmar pinch, she placed each Fruit Loop over a pipe cleaner. Five verbal cues were required for task completion.

A: Heather manipulates tongs well and exhibits a good awareness of positioning of tongs within her hands, which is an indicator that proper scissors use will be attained soon. Good attention to task for entire 25 minutes.

P: Continue prehension activities 3x wk. using a variety of media in 20-30 minute intervals until proper scissors use goal is achieved. Heather will be able to cut a piece of 8 inch x 10 inch paper in half using adaptive spring scissors Ⓘ 3/3 tries by the end of the school year.

Durwood T., OTR/L

Contact Note: Outpatient Clinic – Splint

Date: 9/21/06 **Time**: 1:00 PM Occupational Therapy Note

S: Client states that the splint he was issued last session is not causing any problems. Client also reported that he wore splint "all day at work" for the past 3 days.

O: Client seen in OT clinic for assessment of splint use/tolerance and instruction in ergonomics. Client arrived at clinic wearing Ⓡ cock-up splint. Skin checked following splint removal and no pressure areas noted. Client demonstrated ability to don/doff splint Ⓘ. New stockinette liner issued per client request. Client reported pain in Ⓡ hand ↓ and is now 3/10 (was 6/10 last week). Client was instructed in use of ergonomic equipment (split keyboard and wrist rest) for his job as computer programmer and he was able to demonstrate appropriate use of these devices with splint on. Ergonomic catalog was provided.

A: ↓ pain from 6/10 to 3/10 since wearing splint shows good progress. Client would benefit from continued instruction in ergonomics to enable maximal performance of work tasks.

P: Continue to see client 1x weekly for instruction in ergonomics, median nerve gliding exercises, assessment of splint use and tolerance.

Mary J., COTA
Thomas B., OTR/L

Contact Note: Wheelchair Mobility Instruction

Date: 9/5/06   **Time**: 1400   Occupational Therapy Note

S: Client stated, "I can't wait to try out my new power wheelchair."

O: Client seen 75 minutes in OT clinic for instruction in use of new power w/c. Client was instructed in operating joystick control with Ⓡ hand using wrist stabilization splint. Following skilled instruction, client demonstrated ability to safely navigate w/c around obstacles, turn, and maneuver in tight spaces (i.e., bathroom). Client leans to Ⓛ with posterior pelvic tilt when operating w/c. Preliminary instruction also provided for charging battery and care and maintenance of w/c.

A: Client demonstrates good potential for full Ⓘ in use and care of w/c. He would benefit from Ⓛ lateral w/c support, continued instruction and practice regarding charging battery, and assessment of w/c mobility on uneven surfaces.

P.   Continue OT daily until discharge in 3 days for instruction in use of power wheelchair. By discharge, client will be Ⓘ in w/c mobility outdoors on uneven surfaces and will demonstrate upright posture in w/c c̄ use of appropriate supports.

Richard T., COTA
James F., OTR/L

References

American Psychological Association. (2001). *Publication Manual of the American Psychological Association* (5th ed.). Washington, DC: Author.

American Occupational Therapy Association. (2002). Occupational therapy practice framework: Domain and process. *American Journal of Occupational Therapy, 56*, 609-639.

American Occupational Therapy Association. (2003a). Guidelines for documentation of occupational therapy. *American Journal of Occupational Therapy, 57*, 646-649.

American Occupational Therapy Association. (2003b). Physical agent modalities: A position paper. *American Journal of Occupational Therapy, 57*, 650-651.

American Occupational Therapy Association. (2004a). Guidelines for supervision, roles, and responsibilities during the delivery of occupational therapy services. *American Journal of Occupational Therapy, 58*, 663-667.

American Occupational Therapy Association. (2004b). Scope of practice. *American Journal of Occupational Therapy, 58*, 673-677.

American Occupational Therapy Association. (2005a). Enforcement procedures for the occupational therapy code of ethics. *American Journal of Occupational Therapy, 59*, 643-651.

American Occupational Therapy Association. (2005b). Occupational therapy code of ethics. *American Journal of Occupational Therapy, 59*, 639-642.

American Occupational Therapy Association. (2005c). Standards of practice for occupational therapy. *American Journal of Occupational Therapy, 59*, 663-665.

Centers for Medicare and Medicaid Services. (2003). CMS Medicare Manual System: Pub. 100-8 Program Integrity (Transmittal R43PI). Retrieved December 24, 2005 from http://new.cms.hhs.gov/Transmittals/Downloads/R43PI.pdf

Centers for Medicare and Medicaid Services (2005a). 11 Part B Billing Scenarios for PTs and OTs. Baltimore: Centers for Medicare and Medicaid Services. Retrieved January 4, 2006 from http://www.cms.hhs.gov/TherapyServices/02_billing_scenarios.asp

Centers for Medicare and Medicaid Services. (2005b). HCPCS Level II Codes. Baltimore: Centers for Medicare and Medicaid Services. Retrieved January 12, 2006 from http://www.cms.hhs.gov/MedHCPCSGenInfo/02_HCPCS_LEVEL_II_CODES.asp

Centers for Medicare and Medicaid Services. (2005c). Medicare Benefit Policy Manual (Ch. 15, Section 220.1.2). Baltimore: Centers for Medicare and Medicare Services. Retrieved January 29, 2006 from http://www.cms.hhs.gov/manuals/Downloads/bp102c15.pdf

Centers for Medicare and Medicaid Services. (2005d). Medicare Benefit Policy Manual (Ch. 15, Section 220.1.3). Baltimore: Centers for Medicare and Medicare Services. Retrieved January 29, 2006 from http://www.cms.hhs.gov/manuals/Downloads/bp102c15.pdf

Centers for Medicare and Medicaid Services. (2005e). Medicare Benefit Policy Manual (Ch. 15, Section 220.2). Baltimore: Centers for Medicare and Medicare Services. Retrieved January 13, 2006 from http://www.cms.hhs.gov/manuals/Downloads/bp102c15.pdf

Centers for Medicare and Medicaid Services. (2005f). Overview. Baltimore: Centers for Medicare and Medicaid Services. Retrieved January 4, 2006 from http://www.cms.hhs.gov/MedHCPCSGenInfo/

Clark, G. F. (2005). Developing appropriate student IEP goals. *OT Practice, 10*(14), 12-15.

Coffman-Kadish, N. (2003). Numbering and filing systems. In M. A. Skurka (Ed.), *Health information management: Principles and organization for health information services* (5th ed., pp.105-127). San Francisco: Jossey-Bass.

Fremgen, B.F. (2006). *Medical law and ethics* (2nd ed.). Upper Saddle River, NJ: Pearson Prentice Hall

Gennerman, M. L. (2005). CPT coding: Defining our practice. *OT Practice, 10*(8), 19-23.

Holmquist, B. B. (2004). Incorporating the Occupational Therapy Practice Framework into a mental health practice setting. *Mental Health Special Interest Section Quarterly, 27*(2), 1-4.

Institute for Safe Medication Practices. (2005). ISMP's List of Error- Prone Abbreviations, Symbols, and Dose Designations. Huntingdon Valley, PA: Institute for Safe Medication Practices. Retrieved December 18, 2005 from http://www.ismp.org/

Iyer, P. (2002). Documentation and the allied health professional. In Aiken, T. D. (Ed.), *Legal and ethical issues in health occupations* (pp. 75-96). Philadelphia: W.B. Saunders.

Joint Commission on the Accreditation of Healthcare Organizations. (2005). Questions about Goal #2 (Communication) and the official "do not use" list. Retrieved on December 14, 2005 from http://www.jcaho.org/accredited+organizations/06_goal2_faqs.pdf

Kannenberg, K., & Greene, S. (2003). Infusing occupation into practice: Valuing and supporting the psychosocial foundation of occupation. *OT Practice 8*(10), CE-1-CE-8.

Kettenbach, G. (2004). *Writing SOAP notes with patient/client management formats* (3rd ed.). Philadelphia: F.A. Davis.

Kiger, L. S. (2003). Content and structure of the health record. In M. A. Skurka (Ed.), *Health information management: Principles and organization for health information services* (5th ed., pp. 19-44). San Francisco: Jossey-Bass.

McKelvey, J. (2004). Occupational therapy in acute care hospitals. *OT Practice, 9*(12), CE-1-CE-8.

Merriam-Webster's guide to punctuation and style (2nd ed.). (2001). Springfield, MA: Merriam-Webster.

Olson, J. R. (2004). *Coding and billing for therapy and rehabilitation.* Stillwater, MN: Cross Country Seminars.

Sames, K. M. (2005). *Documenting occupational therapy practice.* Upper Saddle River, NJ: Pearson Prentice Hall.

Shadley, T. S. & Rexrode, A. (2005). Home Health: A journey to improve functional patient outcomes. *OT Practice, 10*(11), CE-1-CE-8.

Slater, D. Y., & Willmarth, C. (2005). Understanding and asserting the Occupational Therapy Scope of Practice. *OT Practice, 10*(19), CE-1-CE-8.

United States Department of Health and Human Services. (2003). Summary of the HIPAA Privacy Rule. Retrieved November 23, 2005 from http://www.hhs.gov/ocr/privacysummary.pdf

World Health Organization. (2006). ICD implementation by countries. Retrieved February 2, 2006 from http://www3.who.int/icd/1.htm

Youngstrom, M. J. (2002a). Introduction to the Occupational Therapy Practice Framework: Domain and process. *OT Practice, 7*(16), CE1-CE-8.

Youngstrom, M. J. (2002b). The Occupational Therapy Practice Framework: The evolution of our professional language. *American Journal of Occupational Therapy, 56*, 607-608.

Resources

American Occupational Therapy Association at www.aota.org

Centers for Medicare and Medicaid Services at www.cms.hhs.gov

Centers for Medicare and Medicaid Services forms at www.cms.hhs.gov/CMSForms

Institute for Safe Medication Practices at www.ismp.org

Joint Commission on Accreditation of Healthcare Organizations at www.jcaho.org

Appendix

Suggestions for Completing the Worksheets

Note to Instructors:

The worksheets in this manual were originally developed for use as in-class exercises. In a classroom situation, students are asked to collaborate on an answer and their collaborative efforts are recorded on a flip chart or blackboard. This is a particularly non-threatening way for students to learn new skills, since it allows them to try out ideas and hear the ideas of others as they work toward a correct result. In this situation the instructor can guide their efforts by asking questions to facilitate good clinical reasoning.

In our experience, many of these exercises do not work as well when used as homework assignments. Because there are so many "correct" ways to complete them, they can be grading nightmares. The suggestions offered here are only a few of the many possible 'good' or "correct" answers. As you do the exercises with a class, you may collect many more equally "good" answers.

Note to Students:

If you are a new OTA using this manual, rather than an instructor, you should be able to work your way through the exercises and check your work against those in this Appendix. Remember that your answer can be different and still be correct, as long as it contains the essential elements. You should not sacrifice your own writing style to be more like someone else's, as long as your information and protocol are essentially correct.

SOAP notes are very difficult to write if there is no treatment session about which to write. Although there are many examples in this manual, there is no substitute for observing or working with actual clients. Only then will you be able to translate your treatment session onto paper in a meaningful way.

Index to Appendix

Chapter 1

Worksheet 1-1: Using the Occupational Therapy Practice Framework

Performance skills related to a clay or craft project might include observable behaviors such as:
activity tolerance, sharing of materials, ability to organize time and materials, sequencing of steps, task initiation, asking for assistance, reaching for objects, sitting upright, speaking with others, gathering and searching for materials, attention to detail, coordination of both hands, pacing of activity, following directions, handling of tools, and many others.

Client factors related to a clay or craft project might include:
UE AROM, strength, vision, hearing, touch, eye-hand coordination, spatial awareness, concept formation, self-esteem, motor planning, gait patterns, muscle tone, stamina, temperament, and many others.

Worksheet 1-2: Occupational Therapy Practice Framework—More Practice

Performance skills related to a cooking task might include behaviors such as:
Knowledge of tools and equipment, carrying objects, adapting to environment, activity tolerance, ability to organize time, materials, and steps, task initiation, clean up, reaching for objects, mobility, lifting, stabilizing, and handling objects, gathering and searching for materials, coordination of both hands, pacing of activity, following directions, and many others.

Client factors related to a cooking task might include:
problem solving, decision making, safety awareness, time management, UE AROM, strength, vision, hearing, smell, touch, eye-hand coordination, spatial awareness, concept formation, motor planning, gait patterns, muscle tone, stamina, temperament, and many others.

Chapter 3

Worksheet 3-1: Using Abbreviations

Translate each sentence written with abbreviations into full English phrases or sentences.

1. Pt. Ⓘ BADL.

   Patient is independent in basic activities of daily living.

2. Client reports ↓ pain Ⓡ shoulder $\bar{p}$ HP.

   Client reports decreased pain in right shoulder after a hot pack treatment.

3. Resident w/c ↔ EOB with SBA.

   Resident transferred from the wheelchair to edge of bed and transferred back to wheelchair with standby assist.

4. Client c/o pain in Ⓡ MCP joint $\bar{p}$ ~ 5 min PROM.

   Client complained of pain in the right metacarpophalangeal joint after approximately 5 minutes of passive range of motion.

5. Client w/c → mat $\bar{c}$ sliding board max Ⓐ x2.

   Client transferred from his wheelchair to the mat using a sliding board and maximum assistance of two people.

6. Pt. O x 4.

   Patient is alert and oriented to person, place, time, and situation.

7. Client has SOB $\bar{c}$ PRE.

   Client has shortness of breath when performing progressive resistive exercises.

8. Pt. has ↓ STM and OCD which limit IADL.

   Patient has decreased short-term memory and obsessive compulsive disorder which limits the ability to perform instrumental activities of daily living.

9. Pt. min Ⓐ AMB bed → toilet 2° ↓ balance.

   Patient requires minimal assistance to ambulate from bed to toilet secondary to decreased balance.

10. Child's FM WFL to don AFO.

    The child's fine motor skills are within functional limits to put on his ankle-foot orthosis.

Worksheet 3-2: Using Abbreviations—Additional Practice

Shorten these notes using only the standard abbreviations in this chapter:

1. Client requires minimal assistance to stand and pull up clothing with partial weight bearing status of left lower extremity.

   Client min Ⓐ to stand and pull up clothing c̄ PWB Ⓛ LE.

2. Patient is able to feed herself independently with use of built-up utensils.

   Pt. Ⓘ feeding c̄ built-up utensils.

3. Client has intact sensation in both upper extremities but complains of minimal pain.

   Client has intact sensation Ⓑ UE but c/o min pain.

4. Client has 55 degrees of passive range of motion in the left index distal interphalangeal joint which is within functional limits.

   55° PROM in Ⓛ DIP is WFL.

5. While sitting on edge of bed, client is able to put on her socks with standby assistance, but requires moderate assistance with putting on and taking off left shoe.

   Client dons socks SBA while sitting EOB but requires mod Ⓐ to don & doff Ⓛ shoe.

6. Student is independent in wheelchair mobility and basic activities of daily living.

   Student Ⓘ w/c mobility and BADL.

7. Patient requires moderate assistance of two people to transfer wheelchair to toilet and from toilet to wheelchair

   Pt. mod Ⓐ x2 w/c ↔ toilet.

8. Patient's toe touch weight bearing status limits her performance of instrumental activities of daily living.

   Pt.'s TTWB limits IADL.

Worksheet 3-3: Deciphering Doctors' Orders and Abbreviations

Translate the following abbreviations into full English phrases or sentences.

1. Dx s/p Ⓡ TKR 2° OA, WBAT
   OT 2x/wk. for BADL, IADL

Diagnosis: status post right total knee replacement secondary to osteoarthritis, weight bearing as tolerated.

Occupational therapy ordered two times weekly for basic and instrumental activities of daily living.

2. X-ray + Ⓛ index finger MC Fx 2° GSW

X-ray is positive for a left index finger metacarpal fracture which is secondary to a gunshot wound.

3. 5 y.o. child has pain 2° bone CA Ⓛ LE

Five-year-old child has pain secondary to bone cancer in left lower extremity.

4. Dx Ⓡ DRUJ Fx c̄ ORIF
    OT 3x/wk. for PAMs PRN, P/AROM, ADL, CPM

 Diagnosis is right distal radioulnar joint fracture with open reduction and internal fixation.

 Occupational therapy ordered three times weekly for physical agent modalities as needed, passive and active range of motion, activities of daily living, and use of continuous passive motion device.

5. 1° Dx PTSD, 2° Dx OCD

  Primary diagnosis is post-traumatic stress disorder, secondary diagnosis is obsessive compulsive disorder.

6. 1° Dx DJD Ⓡ hip, 2° Dx COPD & CHF

Primary diagnosis is degenerative joint disease right hip and secondary diagnosis is chronic obstructive pulmonary disease and congestive heart failure.

7. Dx CAD, TIA

  Diagnosis is coronary artery disease and transient ischemic attack.

Worksheet 3-4: Deciphering Doctors' Orders and Abbreviations—More Practice

Translate the following abbreviations into full English phrases or sentences.

1. Dx PDD-NOS, ADHD
    OT: ADL, SI, FM
    2 x/wk. X 12 wks.

Diagnosis is pervasive developmental disorder not otherwise specified and attention deficit hyperactivity disorder.

Occupational therapy ordered for activities of daily living, sensory integration, fine motor skills.

Twice weekly for twelve weeks.

2. EMG – Ⓡ CTS and - TOS

Electromyogram is negative for right carpal tunnel syndrome and negative for thoracic outlet syndrome.

3. Dx: s/p Ⓛ THR, pt. NWB Ⓛ LE, OOB c̄ walker
    OT eval. and tx.; ADL, Ⓑ UE PREs
    3x/wk. X 4/wks.

Diagnosis is status post left total hip replacement. Patient has non weight bearing status for left lower extremity and may get out of bed with use of walker.

Occupational therapy ordered for evaluation and treatment, activities of daily living, bilateral upper extremity progressive resistive exercises, threes times weekly for four weeks.

4. MRI + TBI, VS stable, BRP

Magnetic resonance imaging is positive for traumatic brain injury. Vital signs are stable, patient is allowed bathroom privileges (able to get out of bed and use the bathroom)

5. CXR – TB but + URI, pt. has DOE and FUO

Chest x-ray is negative for tuberculosis but positive for a upper respiratory infection. Patient has dyspnea upon exertion and fever of unknown origin.

6. Dx. PTSD, ETOH abuse, HBV

Diagnosis is post traumatic stress disorder, alcohol abuse, and hepatitis B virus.

Worksheet 3-5: Additional Practice

Shorten these notes using only the standard abbreviations in this chapter.

1. Pt. seen bedside for instruction in BADL. Max Ⓐ to don LE garments, mod Ⓐ to don UE garments. Mod Ⓐ for bed mobility. Supine → sit min Ⓐ and sit → stand mod Ⓐ.

2. Resident to OT via w/c escort. Resident leans Ⓛ and needs verbal cues and min physical assist to maintain symmetrical posture in midline. Standing pivot transfer w/c → toilet mod Ⓐ for balance. Verbal cues and feedback using a mirror needed to maintain upright posture.

    -or-

    Resident to OT via w/c escort. Resident leans Ⓛ and needs verbal cues and visual feedback from mirror to maintain upright symmetrical posture in midline. Standing pivot w/c → toilet mod Ⓐ for balance.

3. Pt. 10 wks s/p Ⓛ DRUJ Fx and has an URI. Pt. seen in OT clinic for assessment of relevant client factors. Ⓛ shoulder and elbow strength grade 4, wrist strength 3-, grip strength 8#. Light touch intact. Ⓡ UE strength and sensation WFL.

Chapter 4

Worksheet 4-1: Quoting and Paraphrasing

In the following statements, determine which are correct (C) or incorrect (I). Pay close attention to punctuation.

1. **C**   The child stated that she was extremely hungry.
2. **I**   The child stated that "she was starving."
3. **I**   The child "stated I am starving."
4. **C**   The child indicated that she was "starving."
5. **I**   The child stated "I am starving."
6. **I**   The patient asked how to put her splint on?
7. **I**   The patient asked "How do I put my splint on"?
8. **C**   The patient asked about the proper way to put on her splint.
9. **C**   The patient asked, "How do I put my splint on?"
10. **I**   The patient asked "how to put her splint on."
11. **C**   The client requested a new buttonhook.
12. **I**   The client asked if "she could have a new buttonhook."
13. **I**   The client asked, "Can I have a new buttonhook"?
14. **C**   The client asked for a new buttonhook.

15. **C**   The client asked, "Can I have a new buttonhook?"
16. **I**   The client stated "he felt dizzy" as he stood at the kitchen counter.
17. **C**   The client reported feeling "dizzy" while standing at the kitchen counter.
18. **I**   While standing at the kitchen counter, the client stated "he felt dizzy."
19. **I**   The client, while standing at the kitchen counter, stated I feel "dizzy."
20. **C**   The client reported dizziness while standing at the kitchen counter.

Mini-Worksheet 4-2: Spelling

For each of the pairs below, place a check mark next to the word that is spelled correctly.

1. __ defered   ✓ deferred   7. __ recieve   ✓ receive

2. __ definately   ✓ definitely   8. ✓ judgment   __ judgement

3. ✓ dining   __ dinning   9. __ rotator cup   ✓ rotator cuff

4. __ excercise   ✓ exercise   10. __ tolorate   ✓ tolerate

5. __ parrafin   ✓ paraffin   11. __ therapy puddy ✓ therapy putty

6. __ transfering   ✓ transferring   12. ✓ independent   __ independant

Worksheet 4-3: Using Words Correctly

Complete the following sentences by choosing the correct word from the two choices provided in parentheses.

1. The home health **aide** gave the patient a shower. (aid or aide)
2. The client refused to **accept** the doctor's diagnosis. (accept or except)
3. The traumatic brain injury will have a tremendous **effect** on activities of daily living (affect or effect)
4. If the client falls, she probably will **break** her hip due to osteoporosis. (brake or break)
5. The patient became short of **breath** after ambulating to the bathroom. (breath or breathe)
6. The client stated she wanted to **lose** ten pounds. (lose or loose)
7. The patient injured her **dominant** right hand which prevented her from writing. (dominant or dominate)
8. The occupational therapy room is **farther** down the hallway than the physical therapy room. (farther or further)
9. The **current** caseload consists of 10 clients, as compared to 15 clients last week. (currant or current)
10. The OTR asked the patient to **lay** the scissors down on the table. (lay or lie)
11. The weight of the pan was more **than** the patient could manage. (than or then)
12. The clients in the craft group put **their** projects away in the closet. (their or there)
13. The child was able to remain quiet and **stationary** while standing in line. (stationary or stationery)
14. The **principal** of the school attended the IEP meeting. (principal or principle)

Mini-Worksheet 4-4: Capitals

Underline the words that do not correctly follow the rules for capitals.

1. The OTA put the chart on the <u>Physical Therapist's</u> desk.
2. The <u>Patient</u> was going to see his <u>Doctor</u> this afternoon.
3. The OT <u>Aide</u> used <u>velcro</u> and Scotch <u>Tape</u> to fix Mrs. Smith's lapboard during the occupational therapy session.
4. The <u>Doctor</u> spoke to the child who has <u>Chicken Pox</u>.
5. The OTA <u>Student</u> performed a <u>Manual Muscle Test</u> on the client.
6. The client took Tylenol and <u>Antacids</u> before his Rotary Club <u>Meeting</u>.

Mini-Worksheet 4-5: Pronouns, Plurals, Possessives

Look at the following sentences and determine the incorrect components in each sentence. The bolded words indicate the proper corrections.

1. The three **clients'** appointments were all canceled today because their OTA was ill.
2. The **OTA's** lab coat was new.
3. The OTA **student's** resume was reviewed by the OT. –or– The OTA **student's** resume was reviewed by his OT. –or– The OTA **student's** resume was reviewed by her OT.
4. The **child's parents** both attended the therapy session.
5. The children almost hurt **themselves** when they collided with each other in the hallway.
6. The **nurses'** patient gave them all flowers.
7. The **PTs** and **OTs** had the day off.
8. The occupational **therapist's** paperwork was on her desk.
9. One of the **clients** lost **her** splint. –or– One of the **clients** lost **his** splint.

Chapter 5

Worksheet 5-1: Choosing a Subjective Statement

1. In this instance, a pending visit by the client's grandson is not really relevant to the treatment session or to how the client sees her progress. For a different situation it might be important. For example, if the client were planning to go to live with her grandson after discharge, it might be very relevant, and might be a topic the OT wanted to explore further with the client.

2. Even though the client may have been cooperative, and even though it may have been important in this treatment session, it is an assessment of the situation, and does not belong in the "S" category of the note. The client's social conversation might be important in some situations. However, there is a better choice for this particular note.

3. Feeling "pretty good" today might be important, because it might show progress or a change in her condition. In this case, however, it is not the best choice.

4. The client's observations and statements about her upper extremity seem most pertinent to this treatment session. Use of the ® UE is relevant in all aspects of this treatment session.

5. A report of safety concerns by nursing might be relevant to this client's treatment. However, it is not the best choice for the "S" category of this note, for several reasons. A concern by nursing staff should be documented in the nursing notes. The OT should report what she sees, rather than what some other staff member believes. Finally, the subjective section of the SOAP note is used to document the client's views about treatment rather than the staff's views, except in rare instances.

Worksheet 5-2: Writing Concise, Coherent Statements

Client reports using adaptive equipment to don pants and socks while maintaining hip precautions without difficulty. She has no c/o pain with transfers using raised toilet seat. Client states her daughter's home now has the bathroom equipment that was ordered by OT last week.

Chapter 6

Worksheet 6-1: Organizing the "O" With Categories

Some or all of the following categories might be used to make this note easier to read:
Ⓛ UE use or reach/grasp/release
Ⓡ UE use or stabilization for sitting balance
Feeding
Attention/attention to task/attention span
Splint

Depending on the categories selected, the note might read:

Child seen for 60 minutes in daycare setting to work on functional use of Ⓛ UE and feeding skills. Child wore a soft spica thumb splint throughout the treatment session.

Reach/grasp/release:

With min Ⓐ for facilitation of movement of elbow, child demonstrated ability to use Ⓛ UE to reach, grasp and release 5 objects with 1 – 2 verbal cues per object.

Stabilization/Sitting Balance:

Child used Ⓡ UE to stabilize self for unsupported sitting at table.

Feeding:

Child was able to feed self Ⓘ with ~50% spillage, but demonstrated significant limitations in chewing action with ~3 rotary chews and swallowing ~90% of the food without chewing.

Attention: Child required verbal cues throughout the session to maintain attention to task.

Worksheet 6-2: Being More Concise

Client seen in room for skilled instruction in basic self-care activities. Ambulated ~3 ft. to and from shower stall c̄ SBA to manage IV line while ambulating and showering. Shower took ~20 minutes. Client showered and dressed c̄ verbal cues to sit. Client demonstrated good sitting balance but required SBA for balance while standing. Following shower, client assisted back into bed.

-or-

Client seen in room for skilled instruction in safe showering and dressing. Client ambulated ~3' SBA for balance. After verbal cues to sit, client showered in 20 min c̄ SBA to manage IV lines. Dressed upper body Ⓘ while seated and lower body c̄ verbal cues to remain seated.

Chapter 7

Worksheet 7-1: Deemphasizing the Treatment Media

1. Client played a game of catch using bilateral UEs to facilitate grasp and release patterns.

Client worked on functional grasp/release patterns needed to manipulate household objects.

2. Resident put dirt into pot to ½-way point, added seedling, and filled remainder of pot with dirt which was transferred by cup. Resident completed 3 more pots while standing 8 minutes before requiring a 5-minute rest. Resident then resumed standing position for approximately 5 minutes to water completed pots.

Resident demonstrated standing tolerance of 13 minutes with a 5-minute break after 8 minutes in order increase standing balance needed for ADL tasks.

3. Client painted some sungazers in crafts group in order to be able to see that she could do something successfully.

Client completed a series of quick-success projects to increase self-esteem.

Worksheet 7-2: Being Specific About Assist Levels

Without having seen the treatment session, it is impossible to know what part of the tasks required assistance. Here are some suggestions for how the statement might have been worded:

1. Client Supine → sit with min Ⓐ; bed → w/c with mod Ⓐ.

Client supine → sit with min Ⓐ to initiate activity; bed → w/c with mod Ⓐ for balance.

Client supine → sit with min Ⓐ to pull up using trapeze; bed → w/c with mod Ⓐ to lift body weight.

Client supine → sit with min Ⓐ to sequence movement; bed → w/c with mod Ⓐ to bring body to 45°.

Client supine → sit with min Ⓐ swinging legs to EOB; bed → w/c with mod Ⓐ for postural control.

2. Client required SBA in transferring w/c ↔ toilet.

Client required SBA for proper hand placement in transferring w/c ↔ toilet.

Client required SBA to remind him of steps of the transfer when transferring w/c ↔ toilet.

Client required SBA to remind him to lock w/c brakes and lean forward in order to rise from chair.

3. Client retrieved garments from low drawers with min Ⓐ.

Client retrieved garments from low drawers with min Ⓐ to open drawers.

Client retrieved garments from low drawers with min Ⓐ to release trigger on reacher.

Client retrieved garments from low drawers with min Ⓐ to judge halo placement in space.

Client retrieved garments from low drawers with min Ⓐ to grasp handles of drawers.

4. Brushing hair required max Ⓐ.

Brushing hair required max Ⓐ to hold brush.

*Brushing hair required max Ⓐ **to reach back of head.***

*Brushing hair required max Ⓐ **to flex shoulder past 35°.***

5. Client completed dressing, toileting, and hygiene with min Ⓐ.

*Client completed dressing, toileting, and hygiene with min Ⓐ **for sitting balance.***

*Client completed dressing, toileting, and hygiene with min Ⓐ **to reach feet.***

*Client completed dressing, toileting, and hygiene with min Ⓐ **for activities requiring fine motor dexterity.***

*Client completed dressing, toileting, and hygiene with min Ⓐ **to adhere to hip precaution**s.*

Chapter 8

Worksheet 8-1: Justifying Continuing Treatment

Which of the following requires the skill of an occupational therapy assistant?

No   Administering paraffin irrelevant to occupational performance.
Yes   Instructing the client in leisure skills for stress management.
No   Having a client watch a video on assertiveness training without further instruction or without role-playing the techniques.
Yes   Analyzing and modifying functional tasks/activities through the provision of adaptive equipment, or techniques.
Yes   Determining that the modified task is safe and effective.
No   Carrying out a maintenance program.
Yes   Upgrading a strengthening program.
Yes   Teaching the client to use the breathing techniques he has learned while performing his ADL activities.
No   Interpreting initial evaluation results and establishing the intervention plan (This is the responsibility of the OT).
Yes   Providing individualized instruction to the client, family, or caregiver.
No   Giving the patient a replacement piece of hook and loop fastener.
Yes   Providing specialized instruction to eliminate limitations in a functional activity.
Yes   Developing a home program and instructing caregivers.
Yes   Teaching compensatory skills.
No   Gait training.
Yes   Making skilled recommendations to a parent for a child's positioning and feeding.
Yes   Educating clients to eliminate safety hazards.
No   Presenting information handouts (such as energy conservation) without having the client perform the activity.
No   Routine exercise and strengthening programs.
Yes   Adding instruction in lower body dressing techniques to a current ADL program.
Yes   Teaching adaptive techniques such as one-handed shoe tying.

Mini-Worksheet 8-2: Organizing Your Thoughts for Assessment

Problems
- Safety of transferring to and from the toilet.
- Client factors that were not WFL.

Progress/potential
- Verbalized an understanding of safety instructions
- PROM Ⓡ shoulder abduction WNL

Worksheet 8-3: Assessing Factors Not Within Functional Limits

1. Child wrote poorly due to immature pencil grasp and difficulty c̄ spatial orientation of letters.

Poor visuospatial perception and immature pencil grasp interfere with writing skills.

2. Client demonstrated difficulty with balancing her checkbook due to memory and sequencing deficits.

Memory and sequencing deficits cause difficulty c̄ IADL tasks such as balancing checkbook.

3. Client experiencing manic episode and was unable to attend and follow directions for cooking activity.

Client's ↓ process skills 2° manic episode limit performance of IADL tasks

4. Client problem-solved poorly while performing lower body dressing as evidenced by multiple attempts to button pants and don socks.

Client's ↓ ability to problem-solve limits her ability to dress herself s̄ Ⓐ and raises safety concerns in all ADL areas.

Worksheet 8-4: Social Skills Worksheet

What **problems** do you see in the above "S" and "O"?
Unkempt appearance
Interrupts others when talking
Does not stay on topic of conversation

What **areas of occupation** do these problems impact?
Social participation

What evidence of **progress** and/or **potential** do you see?
Engages in conversation
States that she understands the purpose of the group
Willingness to participate in group
Spontaneously shared her ideas and experiences

A: *Client's unkempt appearance, interrupting behaviors, and need for redirection to topic of conversation interfere with her ability to engage in social participation with peers. Her expressed interest in groups, her willingness to engage in conversation and share her ideas show good potential to develop relationships and to express herself verbally in place of acting out. Client would benefit from participating in groups where conversational skills are stressed, from further facilitation of attention to social cues, and from assistance with ADL activities stressing hygiene and appearance.*

Chapter 9

Mini-Worksheet 9-1: Determining the Plan

Continue to treat client 5x wk. for 1 week for skilled instruction in safe transfers and toileting. Home program for AROM and strengthening exercises for Ⓡ shoulder will be taught. Client will be able to Ⓘ demonstrate HEP and will also spontaneously use bilateral grab bars during toilet transfers by the end of next session.

Worksheet 9-2: Completing the Social Skills Plan

P: *Client to be seen daily for the next week to ↑ skills needed for social participation in a variety of contexts. Within 1 week, client will demonstrate ability to engage in a 20 minute conversation without interrupting.*

-or-

P: *Client to continue social skills group 3 X wk and to be given individual feedback daily on her attention to appearance and social cues. By anticipated discharge in 1 week, client will maintain neat appearance and avoid interrupting others in 3/3 one hour group sessions.*

Worksheet 9-3: Completing the Plan: Additional Practice

P.   *Client to continue OT 2 X wk to ↑ functional fine motor skills for BADL. Client will be instructed in one-handed shoe tying technique. By the end of next session client will be Ⓘ in one-handed shoe tying.*

-or-

P.   *Client to continue OT twice weekly for remediation of Ⓡ fine motor skills to enable BADL performance. Client will be instructed in adaptive equipment and by the end of next session will be Ⓘ managing all clothing fastenings.*

Chapter 10

Worksheet 10-1: Mechanics of Documentation

Look at the following contact note and see how many elements you can find that are incorrect or missing. Realize that this note reflects a "special situation" and, therefore, does not need to include the complete S, O, A, and P format.

XYZ School District
Albany, NY

John Doe

3/22/06   Upon arrival to OT room, student reported he had a headache, felt nauseous, and said he was "burning up." OT session defered and student escorted to ~~teach~~ nurse's office.

C. Caring, COTA

1. Time of day not recorded.
2. No health record number or identification number present.
3. Last name is not listed first (may not be required by facility to list last name first).
4. Spaces present without line drawn.
5. Error not corrected properly—should have date and initials above the error.
6. No cosignature (will depend on facility and legal guidelines).
7. Type of note not indicated (contact note).
8. Occupational therapy department not indicated.

9. Spelling error (deferred).
10. OTA's first name only indicated by initial.

Chapter 11

Worksheet 11-1: Evaluating Goal Statements

Determine which of the following goals have all the necessary FEAST components to be useful in occupational therapy documentation. For each goal that is incomplete or inaccurate in some way, indicate what it lacks.

1. By the time of discharge in 2 weeks, client will be able to dress himself with min Ⓐ for balance using a sock aid and reacher while sitting in a wheelchair.

This goal has all the necessary components to be useful.

2. Client will tolerate 15 minutes of treatment daily.

This goal lacks a function and a time frame. In addition, the behavior (tolerating treatment) is not useful because it is not something a client needs to do after discharge. This would be better stated as "tolerate 15 minutes of grooming/hygiene activity."

3. Resident will demonstrate increased coping skills in order to live at home with her granddaughter within 2 weeks.

This goal lacks specificity, and it needs a condition. "Coping skills" is far too broad. The coping skill(s) in question need to be specified.

4. Resident will demonstrate 15 minutes of activity tolerance without rest breaks using Ⓑ UE in order to complete ADL tasks before breakfast each morning.

This goal lacks a time frame, and needs to be turned around to put function first.

Client will be able to complete basic ADL in <15 minutes without rest breaks before breakfast each morning within 2 weeks.

5. In order to be able to toilet self Ⓘ after discharge, client will demonstrate ability to perform a sliding board transfer w/c → mat within the next week.

This goal has all the necessary components to be useful but would be even better if the assist level of the transfer were noted (i.e. Ⓘ)

6. OTA will teach lower body dressing using a reacher, dressing stick and sock aid within 2 tx. sessions.

This goal lacks a proper action and behavior.

7. In order to return to living independently, client will demonstrate ability to balance his checkbook.

This goal lacks a time frame, and would be even better if the assist level for balancing his checkbook were specified (e.g., ability to balance his checkbook Ⓘ).

Worksheet 11-2: Writing Functional, Measurable Goals

Without knowing the client, it is impossible to know what the goal would really be. Here are some suggestions.

1. Your client, Maria, has difficulty with IADL tasks because she is unable to attend to task for more than a few minutes. Since she enjoys cooking and plans to resume cooking after discharge, you have been working with her in the kitchen. You would like to see her able to attend to task for 10 minutes by the time she is discharged next week. Write a goal to increase Maria's attention span.

Client will attend to a cooking activity > 10 minutes without having to be redirected within 3 treatment sessions.

-or-

In order to live ① after discharge, client will demonstrate 10 minute attention span during cooking activity by the end of the 3rd treatment session.

2. Now write a goal for Maria to be able to follow directions so that she can read the back of a boxed meal, and eventually a recipe, when she is cooking.

By anticipated discharge in 1 week, client will complete 3 step written directions for cooking a packaged meal c̄ min. assist.

-or-

Client will demonstrate ability to correctly follow a simple recipe within one week.

3. Bill is having trouble performing dressing tasks after his stroke. In OT you have been teaching him an over-the-head method for putting on his shirt, and have given him a button hook to use. Write a dressing goal for Bill.

Client will be able to don shirt ① using the over-the-head method and a button hook within 2 tx. sessions.

-or-

After skilled instruction, client will be able to dress upper body ① using one handed techniques and adaptive equipment within one week.

4. Susan has significant weakness, and desires to be able to care for her 4-month-old child and also go back to work as a receptionist. Write a goal to increase her activity tolerance. Anticipated discharge is in weeks.

Client will perform >10 minutes of continuous standing activity in order to be able bathe her baby ① by discharge in 2 weeks.

-or-

Within 1 week, client will complete 30 minutes of seated activity without rest breaks in order to return to her job as a receptionist.

5. Alberto wants to live independently in the community, but lacks basic money management skills. Write a goal for Alberto to improve his money management skills.

Client will demonstrate ability to make change ① from $1.00 correctly 3/3 tries within 2 weeks.

-or-

Client will be able to select ads from the newspaper for an apartment that rents for less than 1/3 of his regular monthly income within the next month.

6. Katelyn has become increasingly more depressed over the past several weeks, and was admitted after a suicide attempt. You estimate that you will have her in groups for one week. You would like to see her mood change in that week. Write a goal that will indicate an improved mood.

Within 1 week, client will spontaneously follow her daily schedule, as demonstrated by attending at least 3 scheduled activities per day.

-or-

Client will verbalize an interest in at least one future activity within the next 2 days.

Worksheet 11-3: Writing Functional Measurable Goals: Developmental Disabilities

Without knowing the client, it is impossible to know what the goals should really be. Here are some suggestions for functional goals:

Instrumental ADL—meal preparation:

Client will be able to wash, peel, and chop vegetables to make a salad ① within 4 weeks.

-or-

Within 3 weeks, client will prepare a one step frozen breakfast item using toaster or microwave safely.

Instrumental ADL—household chore:

Client will be able to follow the chore schedule for changing bed sheets within 4 weeks.

-or-

Client will demonstrate ability to set the table ① for 6 place settings within 1 week.

Instrumental ADL—shopping:

In order to ↑ ① in grocery shopping, client will use grocery list to locate 5 items in supermarket with 1 verbal cue for each item within 4 weeks.

-or-

In order to ↑ ① in clothes shopping, client will be able to locate correct size clothing on clothing rack within 2 weeks.

Instrumental ADL—money management/functional math skill:

In order to improve shopping skills, client will use correct denominations to pay cashier ① for items up to $10.00 within 6 weeks.

-or-

Client will select and place correct coins in order to use vending machine ① within 3 weeks.

Communication/Interaction skills:

Client will demonstrate improved social skills by cooperatively playing a simple board game with peers for 20 minutes within 3 weeks.

-or-

Client will demonstrate improved interaction skills by spontaneously allowing roommate to choose T.V. program without an altercation within 3 weeks.

Prevocational skills:

In order to ↑ skills required for employment, client will punch time clock ① 5/5 opportunities within 2 weeks.

-or-

In order to ↑ skills required for employment, client will be able to select appropriate attire for job interview within 2 weeks.

Temporal organization/Time management:

In order to improve time management skills, client will be able to set alarm clock ① within 4 weeks.

-or-

In order to improve time management skills, client will follow daily schedule ① for morning ADL within 1 week.

Chapter 12

Worksheet 12-1: Initial Evaluation Report

Background Data

Criteria	Compliance
Are all of the following present: name, gender, birthdate? Are all applicable diagnoses listed?	Age is given in place of DOB Dx: CVA; R/O OBS 2° Dx: diabetes
Who referred the client to OT, on what date, what services were requested?	Dr. Grantham referred her for evaluation and treatment. No referral date is given.
What is the funding source for this client?	Not noted, but she is 68 which implies Medicare
What length of stay is anticipated for this client?	2 weeks
Why is the client seeking occupational therapy services?	She wants to go home.
Are there any secondary problems, pre-existing conditions, contraindications or precautions that will impact therapy?	Diabetes

Occupational History and Profile

Is there an occupational history/profile? Is it adequate?	There is a brief occupational profile. More information can be obtained during tx.
Which areas of occupation are currently successful and which are problematic?	No successful areas noted. ADL and IADL tasks are problematic.

What factors hinder the client's performance in areas of occupation? What factors support her performance in areas of occupation?	Hinder: ↓ problem solving ability, slow cognitive responses ↓ ability to initiate and sequence tasks. Some client factors not WNL. Support: A nearby daughter who is willing to visit daily and assist with transportation, intact sensation, motor planning and perception WFL, able to stand and transfer with CGA, 1 story home, sedentary hobbies, motivation to go home.
What are the client's priorities? What does she hope to gain from OT?	To go back to her own home
What areas of occupation will be targeted for intervention? Do these match the client's priorities?	ADL and IADL, which do match the client's priorities.
What are the targeted outcomes?	Discharge to home Modified Ⓘ and safety in ADL activities

Results of the Assessment

What types of assessments were used?	Mini-Mental State, ADL evaluation, manual muscle test, sensation, observation, and interview, AROM
What were the results of the assessments?	Results are clearly noted on the evaluation form in the "O".
What client factors, contextual aspects and activity demands are identified as needing attention?	Client factors: ↓ AROM and strength in the Ⓛ UE, ↓ activity tolerance, ↓ problem solving, sequencing, and memory Context: lives alone and daughter unable to provide supervision; needs cues for orientation. Activity demands: Needs cues to initiate and sequence activities and to problem solve.
What factors (strengths, supports) facilitate her occupational performance?	Supportive daughter, client motivated to be Ⓘ
Are there other areas that need to be assessed that are not listed?	Does client use hearing aid, glasses, or ambulation devices? Is there pain, edema, or changes in muscle tone? Other considerations for occupational profile (widowed? spiritual or virtual contexts? habits and routines?)
Is OT appropriate for this client? Why or why not?	Yes—client has good rehab potential to return home and requires OT to improve ADL function

Worksheet 12-2: Intervention Plan

Criteria	Compliance
Are specific OT interventions identified?	Yes
Are the intervention goals and objectives measurable and realistic?	Yes
Are the goals and objectives directly related to the client's occupational role performance?	Yes
What is the anticipated frequency/duration of services?	45 minute sessions 5X wk for 2 weeks.
What is the discontinuation criteria or expected outcomes?	Ability to live at home safely without supervision
What is the anticipated discharge location?	Home
What is the anticipated plan for follow-up care?	Not noted
Where will services be provided?	XYZ Hospital as inpatient

Mini-Worksheet 12-4: Choosing Activities—More Practice

How would you work on these goals at the same time? What would your treatment activities be?

1. Student will be able to Ⓘ open all lunch containers and wrappers.
2. Student will spontaneously use Ⓛ hand as a functional assist for bimanual classroom tasks 5/5 opportunities.
3. Student will attend to classroom tasks for 10 minute periods with only 1 verbal cue for redirection.

You can work with the child at lunchtime in the cafeteria or in another room. You may have the child try to open all the lunch items such as: lunch box, brown bag, milk container, sandwich wrapper, plastic containers, snack bags/wrappers, etc. You will note if the child is spontaneously incorporating use of both hands for these tasks and how well the Ⓛ hand is being used as a functional assist for setting up lunch items. You will also note the number of minutes for attention to task and if child needs to be redirected to task.

-or-

You might also have the child perform another task that involves opening containers, such as a craft project where materials are in snack bags or small jars/containers. Again, you would note Ⓛ hand use and attention span.

Chapter 13

Worksheet 13-1: Treatment, Visit, or Contact Notes

Criteria	Compliance
Is client information (name, gender, birthdate, diagnosis, precautions and/or contraindications) present?	No date of birth or diagnosis given. In an acute care setting the client information is commonly stamped onto each page of the health record with an addressograph card. No precautions or contraindications given.
What is the date and time of the contact?	4/14/06 at 8:30 AM
What is the type of contact?	Client contact for ADL interventions

What are the names and positions of the person's involved in the contact?	John B., client Bonnie B, COTA
Is there a summary of the intervention or the information communicated during the contact?	Yes
Is the client's participation in the contact (or the reason service was missed) indicated?	Yes
Is there an indication that the task or environment was modified or that adaptive or assistive devices were used or fabricated?	Client required set up of task, no adaptations in this intervention.
Is there an indication of any consultation/education/training and the persons involved?	Client instructed in ADL and needs instruction in energy conservation.

Worksheet 13-2: Progress Notes

Criteria	Compliance
Is client information (name, date of birth, gender, diagnosis, precautions and/or contraindications) present?	No. Name and record number would be stamped by addressograph or written on each page. Since this is an inpatient health record, the other information would not necessarily be written by the therapist onto each progress note sheet.
What is the frequency of services? How long have services been provided?	8 groups per week offered; client attended 6/8. The note covers one week. SOC not noted.
What techniques and strategies were used? Was the client or caregiver provided with programs or any training?	Assertion group; communication group; IADL group. No training to caregivers as yet; client to talk to husband about leisure plans
Were any environmental or task modifications provided? Were any orthotic devices or adaptive equipment provided?	Client needs structure
What other pertinent client updates are given?	Leisure plan to be developed and discussed with husband and social worker; goals updated
What is the client's response to occupational therapy services?	Shares without prompting; spontaneously answered a question; offered to help a peer; increased attention to appearance; unprompted attendance.
What progress is the client making toward her goals?	Two goals met, one goal continued, one goal discontinued. Progress as noted above
What areas of occupation are being addressed?	Social participation, IADL, self-care, leisure
What recommendations are made and why? What is the client's input regarding continuation of the intervention plan or any changes needed?	Plan structured day to prevent relapse; attend groups 2 more days. Leisure plan recommended; no notation of client's input to changes

Worksheet 13-3: Reevaluation Reports

Criteria	Compliance
Is there any new information about the client's medical condition or occupational profile?	Pain has decreased, ergonomic keyboard used at work
What was the purpose of the reevaluation?	Determination of continued need for occupational therapy services
What assessments were used initially? What assessments are used now?	ADL/IADL interview, goniometry; grip strength; interview, visual inspection for edema
How do the results compare with the previous evaluation results?	Improvement in client factors, ADL, IADL and work status. Decrease in pain.
What occupational changes are evident? In what ways has the client made progress?	Able to do more ADL, IADL and work tasks successfully. Obtained ergonomically shaped keyboard
Are there areas of occupation that are still problematic?	Still has difficulty with locked doors; some client factors still not WNL
What changes in occupational therapy treatment, goals, or referrals will be made as a result of the reevaluation?	Services will be discontinued

Worksheet 13-4: Transition Plan

Criteria	Compliance
What is the client's occupational performance at this time?	At a 4 month level, working on reach, grasp, and release, rolling, ability to sustain anti-gravity positions. Visual regard, midline orientation, and visually directed reach are problematic.
What is the current setting?	Birth-to-Three program
What will the new setting be?	Preschool program
What is the reason for the transition?	Age
When will the transition occur?	May (1 month)
What activities will occur throughout the transition plan?	Home program
What recommendations are made for occupational therapy services in the new setting?	Reevaluate; continue OT, PT, and speech therapy
What other recommendations, equipment, or follow-up are indicated in this plan?	None noted

Worksheet 13-5: Discharge Summary

Criteria	Compliance
Is information present about the client's medical condition? How has the condition changed?	No
What was the initial date of OT service? What was the end date of OT service? Are number of intervention sessions listed?	9/25/06 10/19/06 20 sessions
What types of interventions were provided? What was the client's progress toward goals?	Interventions: ADL instruction, adaptive equipment, adaptive techniques, HEP, improvement of client factors (strength) in independence Met all treatment goals

What was the client's beginning and ending status regarding ability to engage in occupations?	Beginning: Mod Ⓐ for ADL task except for max Ⓐ in bathing. Ending: SBA for all ADL tasks, except Ⓘ in toileting
Was the client satisfied with outcomes?	Pleased (in SOAP format) Not given in facility format
What recommendations or follow-up are listed? How well do they pertain to the future needs of the client?	Continue HEP Outpatient physical therapy, 2 pieces of adaptive equipment and home modifications recommended for safety and Ⓘ

Chapter 15

Worksheet 15-1: SOAPing Your Note

Indicate beside each of the following statements under which section of the SOAP note you would place it.

O   Client supine → sit in bed Ⓘ.

O   Client moved kitchen items from counter to cabinet Ⓘ using Ⓛ hand.

S   Parent reports child's handwriting has significantly improved within the past month.

A   Problems include decreased coordination, strength, sensation, and proprioception in left hand which create safety risks in home management tasks.

S   Client reports that his fingers are stiff this morning and that he is having trouble handling small items like buttons.

P   By the end of next treatment session, client will be Ⓘ donning/doffing splint.

A   Client's ↑ of 15 minutes in activity tolerance for UE activities permits her to prepare a light meal Ⓘ.

O   Child seen in OT clinic to promote development of FM skills for BADL.

P   In order to return to work, client will demonstrate an increase of 10 lbs. grasp in Ⓛ hand by 1/3/07.

A   Decreased proprioception and motor planning limit client's ability to dress upper body.

P   Continue retrograde massage to Ⓡ hand for edema control.

A   Client's correct identification of inappropriate positioning 100% of the time would indicate memory WFL.

P   Consumer will be seen 2X weekly to improve task behaviors in order to obtain a job.

S   Client reports that she cannot remember her hip precautions.

A   Client would benefit from further instruction to incorporate total hip precautions into lower body dressing, bathing, and hygiene.

A   Learning was evident by client's ability to improve with repetition.

A   Client's request to take rest breaks demonstrates knowledge of her limitations in endurance.

O   Client required 3 verbal prompts to interact with peers in OT social group.

A   3+ muscle grade of extension in Ⓡ wrist extensors this week shows good progress toward goals.

O   Client completed weight shifts of trunk x10 in each of anterior, posterior, left and right lateral directions in preparation for standing to perform home management tasks.

A   Poor temporal organization interferes with getting to work on time.

Worksheet 15-2: Writing the S—Subjective

Pt reports significant arthritis in Ⓡ shoulder and knee, and prefers to approach transfers from the affected side. Pt. reports, "It hurts to bear weight on my leg." Pt also stated w/c → bed sliding board transfers are the most difficult, and reported fatigue after transfer.

-or-

Client reports arthritis is Ⓡ shoulder and knee and pain bearing weight on Ⓡ LE. Pt able to verbalize needs regarding transfer (placement of board and approach from affected side). Client reports fatigue after transfer.

Worksheet 15-3: Making Opening Lines Better

1. Client practiced laundry tasks for 45 minutes.

Client seen in room for 45 minutes to increase Ⓘ in IADL activities, to decrease safety concerns during functional mobility, and to provide instruction on proper use of adaptive equipment for home management tasks.

-or-

Client seen in hospital room for 45 minutes for education on use of adaptive equipment to safely perform home management tasks.

-or-

Client seen in OT room for 45 minutes for education on safety concerns during IADL and skilled instruction in use of adaptive equipment for laundry tasks.

-or-

Client seen in OT clinic for 45 minutes for skilled instruction in use of adaptive equipment and hip precaution education during performance of home management tasks.

2. Consumer seen at workshop for one hr. to improve job skills.

Consumer seen at workshop for 1 hr. to address time management, cognitive, sensory and bilateral integration barriers to performing work tasks effectively.

-or-

Consumer seen at workshop for 1 hr. to work on sequencing, bilateral coordination, concentration and time management skills while completing work task of package handling.

-or-

Consumer seen at workshop for 1 hr. to improve time management and sequencing skills, increase bilateral coordination and decrease distractibility at work.

-or-

Consumer seen @ workshop for 1 hr. for skilled instruction in task sequencing, bilateral coordination and techniques to improve time management and decrease distractibility for job skills.

3. Client seen in his hospital room bedside for 30 minutes for feeding.

Client seen bedside for 30 minutes for instruction in adaptive equipment for feeding and perceptual remediation.

-or-

Client seen bedside for 30 minutes to increase Ⓘ self feeding and to decrease Ⓛ neglect.

-or-

Client seen bedside for 30 minutes to instruct client in compensatory methods for feeding and to ↑ awareness of left side.

-or-

Client seen at bedside for 30 minutes to provide skilled instruction in self feeding methods and improve perceptual skills.

4. Worked with client in kitchen for 1 hr. to ↑ ① in cooking.

Client seen in kitchen for 1 hr. to increase activity tolerance for standing and increase awareness of affected UE for safety in cooking.

-or-

Client seen in kitchen for 1 hr. to address safety concerns regarding standing tolerance and Ⓛ UE neglect.

-or-

Client seen in kitchen for 1 hr. to increase activity tolerance for standing and ↑ attention affected UE to increase safety while cooking.

-or-

Client seen in kitchen for 1 hr. to work on cooking tasks with attention to standing tolerance, affected UE position, and safety.

-or-

Client seen in kitchen for 1 hr. for skilled instruction in kitchen safety to improve standing tolerance and attention to affected UE.

Worksheet 15-4: Writing the "O"—Objective

1. First, an opening line is needed stating where, for how long, and for what purpose the client was seen. One possibility is:

Client seen in room for skilled instruction in ADL tasks and assessment of splinting needs.

-or-

Client seen bedside for skilled instruction in compensatory dressing techniques and assessment of splinting needs.

2. Second, the categories could be reduced to 3 (toileting, dressing, and splinting assessment) or 2 (BADL and splinting assessment).
3. Third, it would be helpful to know what part of the task needed assistance.
4. Fourth, the UE and LE wording is not inclusive enough, since the client is dressing the upper and lower body rather than just the extremities. Specific types of clothing are not indicated (i.e., elastic waist paints, turtleneck sweater).
5. Finally, under "hand status" there is no functional component, and "index finger greatest amount" is not very informative.

Worksheet 15-5: Differentiating between Observations and Assessments

O   Client is unable to don Ⓛ LE prosthesis for functional mobility.

A   Inability to don Ⓛ LE prosthesis Ⓘ prevents client from performing safe functional mobility around the house to live alone.

A   Decreased tolerance to auditory stimuli limit's the student's ability to attend to classroom tasks.

O   Student requires verbal cues to stay on task due to decreased tolerance to auditory stimuli.

O   Client was unable to incorporate relaxation and stress reduction techniques, requiring several verbal prompts to complete task.

A   Inability to incorporate relaxation and stress reduction techniques when interacting with sales clerk limits her ability to Ⓘ manage shopping tasks p̄ discharge.

Reword the following observations to make them assessments.

1. Client demonstrated difficulty with balancing checkbook due to memory and sequencing deficits.

Decreased memory and sequencing abilities limit client's ability to perform IADL activities such as financial management tasks.

-or-

Memory and sequencing deficits interfere with client's ability to perform IADL such as financial management tasks, and limit her ability to return to an Ⓘ living situation.

-or-

Deficits in memory and sequencing limit the client's ability to do many IADL, for example, balancing her checkbook.

-or-

Deficits in memory and sequencing lead to difficulty with IADL tasks such as financial management tasks necessary for household management.

2. Client unable to complete homemaking tasks or basic self-care activities independently due to Ⓛ neglect, impulsive behavior, and decreased attention to task.

Decreased safety awareness, poor attention, and perceptual deficits limit client's ability to complete homemaking tasks and self-care activities Ⓘ.

-or-

Decreased safety awareness and inattention to Ⓛ side interfere with client's ability to complete homemaking tasks and decrease ability to successfully complete basic self-care activities Ⓘ.

-or-

Decreased safety awareness and cognitive and perceptual deficits prevent client from performing homemaking and BADL Ⓘ and safely.

3. After the use of behavior modification techniques, child demonstrated ability to remain seated at desk for the remainder of the treatment session.

You could take a positive or a negative approach to this one.

Positive:

Child's ability to remain seated at desk with the aid of behavior modification techniques indicates good potential for improving problem behaviors in school.

-or-

Child's positive response to behavior modification techniques shows good potential to meet classroom behavior goals.

Negative:

The need for behavior modification techniques to remain seated at desk limit child's ability to succeed with academic tasks.

-or-

Client's need for instruction in behavior modification limits his ability to concentrate effectively in classroom situations.

Worksheet 15-6: Problems, Progress, and Rehab Potential

Problems:
After reading through this note, several problems stood out for this OTA:

- Dynamic sitting balance
- Weight shifting
- Posture
- Transfers

(The four above are related to safety and functional mobility.)

- Decreased AROM in Ⓡ UE (mod Ⓐ to reach)
- Cognition

On thinking a little further, the OTA decided that the "cognition" problem might really be one of the following, since the client does seem to understand the goal of the activity.

- Short-term memory
- Motor planning
- Problem solving
- Initiation

Finally, the OTA decides that the problem with initiation is probably some combination of problem solving and motor planning deficit.

Progress/Rehab Potential/Strengths
Ability to understand the treatment goal

The OTA then groups the problems according to the impact they have on the client's occupational performance. The OTA decides that the first three cause difficulty with functional mobility, and are of particular concern because they create safety issues. The motor planning and initiation problem is a concern in the area of self care, as is the problem with decrease in AROM of the right UE. The need for continual instruction, whether it is a problem with short term memory or with his ability to problem solve, is likely to require a lot of attention from a caregiver at home. The client does, however, understand why he is doing the given task. As long as the goals are not set too high, the client should be able to make good progress in rehabilitation. The OTA's assessment and plan read as follows:

A: Deficits in postural control, dynamic sitting balance, and weight shifting raise safety concerns when transferring. ↓ AROM and motor planning ability negatively impact ability to perform self-care tasks. A need for continual instruction to prevent unsafe performance of ADL tasks requires a high level of caregiver assistance. Client's ability to understand treatment goal indicates good rehab potential for the goals established. Client would benefit from continued skilled instruction in activities to ↑ balance, safe functional mobility, and Ⓘ in ADL tasks.

P: Continue tx. daily for 3 weeks for skilled instruction in self care tasks and safe transfers. In 3 weeks client will be able to transfer safely from wheelchair to bed or toilet c̄ min Ⓐ for balance.

Another OTA might assess the session a little differently. For example:

A: Problems include deficits in motor planning, movement initiation, cognition, and muscle weakness in Ⓡ UE which ↓ safety in ADL tasks and functional mobility. Activity tolerance has improved since yesterday from < 1 minute to >3 minutes without a rest break. Client would benefit from skilled OT to increase balance, functional mobility, and grasp/release activities with involved UE in order to ↑ Ⓘ in self-care activities.

P: Continue tx. twice daily for ½ hour sessions to work on Ⓡ UE movement and cognitive retraining in order to complete grooming activities with min Ⓐ. Client will be able to place toothpaste on toothbrush with min Ⓐ by the end of next tx. session.

-or-

A: Decreased functional use of the Ⓡ UE, decreased sitting balance, and difficulty with sequencing and problem solving limit ability to perform ADL. Increased shoulder flexion and improved motor planning since initial evaluation and increased understanding of treatment activities would indicate good rehab potential. Client would benefit from continued skilled OT to increase functional AROM, exercises in grasp, exercises in weight shifting to improve dynamic sitting balance, and evaluation of both cognitive status and ability to initiate activity in order to increase Ⓘ in ADL tasks.

P: Continue OT twice daily for 30 minute sessions for 2 weeks to increase dynamic sitting balance in preparation for ADL training. Client will be able to reach for grooming items placed slightly beyond arm's reach c̄ CGA within 1 week.

Worksheet 15-7: The "Almost" Note

Here we have a note that seems good on the surface, but demonstrates some problems in critical thinking. The most outstanding problem with this note is that the OTA is mixing her "O" data and her "A" data.

1. First, it would have helped the "S" if the OTA had asked pertinent questions, such as what the client's pain levels were.

2. Second, there is nothing in the "O" to show that skilled occupational therapy is being provided. The list of observations of assist levels fails to provide the richness of the skill used in treatment. The OTA erroneously puts some of that information in the "A" section, rather than assessing the data. In the "A" the OTA tells us:

Client Ⓘ in dressing while sitting EOB, but is min Ⓐ in dressing when standing with a walker. Ⓛ UE AROM is WFL but Ⓡ UE has deficits noted in shoulder flexion. Client SBA in bed mobility when rolling to unaffected side and min Ⓐ in sit → stand 2° to ↓ UE strength. Client SBA for transfer to unaffected side in pivot transfer bed → w/c and min Ⓐ w/c → toilet.

Even in this information were moved into the "O", there is nothing to tell us what part of the task the assistance was for. The OTA uses a non-standard abbreviation "VC's". She means verbal cues, but since VC is a standard health term meaning vital capacity, it is inappropriate in its usage here and is not on the "approved" list in this manual.

3. Third, the coordination deficits mentioned in the "A" section come out of the blue. There is no mention of coordination in the opening statement "...for work on dressing and functional mobility" nor is it mentioned as a problem in the "O". Thus the statement that coordination deficits are one of the problems noted and the statement that the client would benefit from coordination exercises are unsubstantiated. Remember not to introduce any new information in the "A" section of your note. Information regarding transfers and bed mobility is redundant because it is simply stated twice without any additional assessment or clinical judgment. There is no real assessment of the meaning of the data found in the "S" and the "O." There is a short list of problem areas, but no assessment of their impact of ability to engage in meaningful occupation, and no assessment of the rehab potential shown by the client's willingness to "do whatever it takes to get out of the hospital."

The best thing for this OTA to do is to rewrite the "O" section, providing a more comprehensive picture of the treatment session. Then she needs to assess the data based on skilled observations and clinical reasoning. There needs to be an indication of how the observed data impacts the occupational performance of the client, before the statements about what the client would benefit from.

Depending on the assessment the OTA makes, the plan to work on balance may be appropriate, or it may be only one of the things to be addressed.

Worksheet 15-8: Writing Functional and Measurable Goals

Client will pivot while standing with SBA during toilet transfers in 1 day.
- Reword this goal for clarity. For example:

Client will be able to perform standing pivot transfer to toilet SBA for safety within 1 day.

-or-

Client will be able to transfer w/c → toilet standing pivot SBA within one day.

Client will be min Ⓐ in dressing UE and LE in 10 days.
- This goal needs to be written in terms of what the client needs, rather than stating that he will be a particular assist level. It is a small item that shows more respect to word the goal statement so that it acknowledges that the client is more than his ability to dress himself.
- Specify the conditions under which the client will dress himself (including what parts of the task need assistance), rather than that he will dress only his upper and lower extremities. For example:

Client will be able to dress self sitting EOB with min Ⓐ to pull pants over hips within 10 days.

-or-

Within 10 days, client will dress self with modified Ⓘ using a dressing stick and long shoehorn.

-or-

Client will dress self with min Ⓐ for balance within 10 days while adhering to 100% of hip precautions.

Deemphasizing the Treatment Media

Client will place 8 half-inch screws and washers on a block of wood with holes by next treatment session.

By the end of 2nd treatment session, client will demonstrate ability to handle small objects needed to return to work by placing 8 half-inch screws into a block of wood in < 5 minutes.

Client will make a clock using the appropriate materials by anticipated discharge in one week.

Pt will demonstrate the ability to grasp/place/release objects of various sizes needed for IADL activities by anticipated discharge in 2 weeks.

-or-

Client will demonstrate ability to follow written directions for IADL tasks by assembling a clock from written instructions within one week.

Client will stay in his chair without reminders and spend at least 30 minutes lacing the leather billfold during the 45 minute craft group session in 2 weeks.

Within 1 month, client will demonstrate attention to task needed to qualify for sheltered workshop program by staying in his chair without reminders and attending to craft project for 30 minutes or more.

Index

WAIT

...There's More!

SLACK Incorporated's Health Care Books and Journals offers a wide selection of products in the field of Occupational Therapy. We are dedicated to providing important works that educate, inform and improve the knowledge of our customers. Don't miss out on our other informative titles that will enhance your collection.

Ryan's Occupational Therapy Assistant: Principles, Practice Issues, and Techniques, Fourth Edition
Karen Sladyk, PhD, OTR/L, FAOTA; Sally Ryan, COTA, ROH
624 pp., Soft Cover, 2005, ISBN 10: 1-55642-740-9,
ISBN 13: 978-1-55642-740-4, Order# 37409, **$58.95**

To help OTAs keep pace with the latest developments in occupational therapy, Sally Ryan and Karen Sladyk present a new edition of the classic Ryan's *Occupational Therapy Assistant: Principles, Practice Issues, and Techniques.* This updated Fourth Edition integrates the *Occupational Therapy Practice Framework: Domain and Process* throughout each section, while including evidence-based practice and research to support the treatment options presented.

OTA Exam Review Manual, Second Edition
Karen Sladyk, PhD, OTR/L, FAOTA
224 pp., Soft Cover, 2005, ISBN 10: 1-55642-701-8,
ISBN 13: 978-1-55642-701-5, Order# 37018, **$33.95**

The *OTA Exam Review Manual* is now available in a completely updated and revised second edition with over 550 questions. This invaluable study tool is designed to guide students through the studying process from start to finish. With a redesigned question format to match the NBCOT exam, more questions, and an on-line testing component, this second edition is a study guide that inspires critical thinking.

The OTA's Guide to Writing SOAP Notes, Second Edition
Sherry Borcherding, MA, OTR/L; Marie J. Morreale, OTR/L
200 pp., Soft Cover, 2007, ISBN 10: 1-55642-779-4,
ISBN 13: 978-1-55642-779-4, Order# 37794, **$31.95**

Quick Reference Dictionary for Occupational Therapy, Fourth Edition
Karen Jacobs, EdD, OTR/L, CPE, FAOTA; Laela Jacobs, OTR
600 pp., Soft Cover, 2004, ISBN 10: 1-55642-656-9,
ISBN 13: 978-1-55642-656-8, Order# 36569, **$26.95**

Management Skills for the Occupational Therapy Assistant
Amy Solomon, OTR; Karen Jacobs, EdD, OTR/L, CPE, FAOTA
176 pp., Soft Cover, 2003, ISBN 10: 1-55642-538-4,
ISBN 13: 978-1-55642-538-7, Order# 35384, **$35.95**

Documentation Manual for Writing SOAP Notes in Occupational Therapy, Second Edition
Sherry Borcherding, MA, OTR/L
256 pp., Soft Cover, 2005, ISBN 10: 1-55642-719-0,
ISBN 13: 978-1-55642-719-0, Order# 37190, **$33.95**

Foundations of Pediatric Practice for the Occupational Therapy Assistant
Amy Wagenfeld, PhD, OTR/L; Jennifer Kaldenberg, MSA, OTR/L
400 pp., Soft Cover, 2005, ISBN 10: 1-55642-629-1,
ISBN 13: 978-1-55642-629-2, Order# 36291, **$44.95**

OT Study Cards in a Box, Second Edition
Karen Sladyk, PhD, OTR/L, FAOTA
255 pp Cards w/Carrier, 2003, ISBN 10: 1-55642-620-8,
ISBN 13: 978-1-55642-620-9, Order# 36208, **$44.95**

The Successful Occupational Therapy Fieldwork Student
Karen Sladyk, PhD, OTR/L, FAOTA
240 pp., Soft Cover, 2002, ISBN 10: 1-55642-562-7,
ISBN 13: 978-1-55642-562-2, Order# 35627, **$38.95**

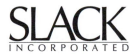

A Quick Checklist for Evaluating Your Note

Use the following summary chart as a quick reference guide to be sure that your note contains all the essential elements.

S: Subjective

☐ 1. Use something significant the client says about his treatment or condition

O: Objective

☐ 1. Begin this section with length of time, where and for what the client was seen.

☐ 2. Report what you see, either chronologically or using categories,

☐ 3. Remember to do the following:
- Deemphasize the media
- Specify what the part of the task the assistance was for
- Show skilled OT happening
- Leave yourself out
- Focus on the client's response
- Avoid being judgmental

A: Assessment

☐ 1. Look at the data in your "O" sentence by sentence, asking yourself what problems, progress, and rehab potential you see.

☐ 2. Ask yourself "So what?" Why is this important in the client's life? For each underlying factor not within functional limits, identify the impact it will have on an area of occupation

☐ 3. End the "A" with "client would benefit from..."
- Justify continued skilled OT
- Set up the plan

(Be sure the time lines and activities you are putting in your plan match the skilled OT you say your client needs.)

P: Plan

☐ 1. Specify how often the client will be seen and for how long.

☐ 2. Tell what you will be working on during that time

☐ 3. End with a LTG or STG, whichever is more appropriate for your client & practice setting

☐ Make certain engagement in occupation is integral to the note.

☐ Make certain everything goes together. For example, if you talk about inability to dress in the problem list, don't switch to feeding in the goals and showering in the plan.

☐ Remember to sign and date your note.

If you have read the text carefully you will understand what each item means. For a more complete explanation, refer to the chapter that provides information in detail. There is a brief explanation of SOAP guidelines on the back of this sheet.

From Borcherding S, Morreale M. *The OTA's Guide to Writing SOAP Notes, Second Edition.* © 2007 SLACK Incorporated.

"S" Subjective

☐ Use something significant the client says about his treatment or condition.

☐ If there is nothing significant, ask yourself whether you are using your interview skills to elicit the information about how the client sees things.

"O" Objective

☐ Begin this section with length of time, where the client was seen and for what reason. For example:
Client seen for 30 minutes bedside for functional mobility

☐ Report what you see, either chronologically or using categories.

☐ Remember to do the following:

   ☐ Focus on performance elements & deemphasize the media. For example:
   Client worked on tripod pinch using pegs.

   ☐ When giving assist levels, specify the part of the task the assistance was for.
   Client min Ⓐ for correct hand placement during pivot transfer to toilet.

   ☐ Show skilled OT happening—make it clear that you were not just a passive observer.
   For example, don't just list all the assist levels and think that is enough.

   ☐ Write from the client's point of view, leaving yourself out.
   Client repositioned rather than *OTA repositioned the client.*

   ☐ Focus on the client's response, rather than on what you did.
   Client able to don socks using dressing stick after demonstration.

   ☐ Avoid being judgmental.
   For example, say client "*...didn't complete the activity.*" Don't add " *...because he was stubborn.*"

"A" Assessment

☐ Look at the data in your "O" sentence by sentence, identifying problems, progress, and rehab potential. Ask yourself what each statement means for the client's occupational performance. This is your assessment of the data. For example, if in your "O" you noted that client falls to the left when sitting unsupported, what do you think this means he will be unable to do for himself? For example: *Client unable to sit EOB unsupported to dress.*

☐ Be sure you have not introduced any new information.

☐ End the "A" with "client would benefit from..."

☐ Justify continued skilled OT: *Client would benefit from skilled instruction in energy conservation techniques as well as continued work on AROM of the UEs, strengthening, and compensatory techniques for performing IADL tasks one handed.*

☐ Set-up the plan. (Be sure the time lines you are putting in your plan match the skilled OT you document that your client needs.) For example, if you justify skilled OT by saying only, *Client would benefit from skilled instruction in energy conservation techniques*, then do not say that you plan to treat him twice a day for 2 weeks. Skilled instruction in energy conservation should take only one session, or at most two sessions.

"P" Plan

☐ Specify frequency and duration of treatment: *Continue tx. one hour daily for 2 weeks.*

☐ Identify the specific performance areas that will be addressed during that time: *Client to continue OT one hour daily for 2 weeks for instruction in Ⓘ in bathing, grooming, and hygiene.*

☐ End with a LTG or STG, whichever is more appropriate for your client and the practice setting: *By the end of the week, client will be able to don socks Ⓘ sitting EOB without losing balance.*

From Borcherding S, Morreale M. *The OTA's Guide to Writing SOAP Notes, Second Edition.* © 2007 SLACK Incorporated.